MICHAEL GROSSMAN

THE CITY UNIVERSITY OF NEW YORK

THE DEMAND FOR HEALTH:

A THEORETICAL AND EMPIRICAL

INVESTIGATION

OCCASIONAL PAPER 119

NATIONAL BUREAU OF ECONOMIC RESEARCH

NEW YORK 1972

Distributed by COLUMBIA UNIVERSITY PRESS

NEW YORK AND LONDON

For Ilene who induced me
to "choose" a long life

Relation of the Directors to the Work and Publications of the National Bureau of Economic Research

1. The object of the National Bureau of Economic Research is to ascertain and to present to the public important economic facts and their interpretation in a scientific and impartial manner. The Board of Directors is charged with the responsibility of ensuring that the work of the National Bureau is carried on in strict conformity with this object.

2. The President of the National Bureau shall submit to the Board of Directors, or to its Executive Committee, for their formal adoption all specific proposals for research to be instituted.

3. No research report shall be published until the President shall have submitted to each member of the Board the manuscript proposed for publication, and such information as will, in his opinion and in the opinion of the author, serve to determine the suitability of the report for publication in accordance with the principles of the National Bureau. Each manuscript shall contain a summary drawing attention to the nature and treatment of the problem studied, the character of the data and their utilization in the report, and the main conclusions reached.

4. For each manuscript so submitted, a special committee of the Board shall be appointed by majority agreement of the President and Vice Presidents (or by the Executive Committee in case of inability to decide on the part of the President and Vice Presidents), consisting of three directors selected as nearly as may be one from each general division of the Board. The names of the special manuscript committee shall be stated to each Director when the manuscript is submitted to him. It shall be the duty of each member of the special manuscript committee to read the manuscript. If each member of the manuscript committee signifies his approval within thirty days of the transmittal of the manuscript, the report may be published. If at the end of that period any member of the manuscript committee withholds his approval, the President shall then notify each member of the Board, requesting approval or disapproval of publication, and thirty days additional shall be granted for this purpose. The manuscript shall then not be published unless at least a majority of the entire Board who shall have voted on the proposal within the time fixed for the receipt of votes shall have approved.

5. No manuscript may be published, though approved by each member of the special manuscript committee, until forty-five days have elapsed from the transmittal of the report in manuscript form. The interval is allowed for the receipt of any memorandum of dissent or reservation, together with a brief statement of his reasons, that any member may wish to express; and such memorandum of dissent or reservation shall be published with the manuscript if he so desires. Publication does not, however, imply that each member of the Board has read the manuscript, or that either members of the Board in general or the special committee have passed on its validity in every detail.

6. Publications of the National Bureau issued for informational purposes concerning the work of the Bureau and its staff, or issued to inform the public of activities of Bureau staff, and volumes issued as a result of various conferences involving the National Bureau shall contain a specific disclaimer noting that such publication has not passed through the normal review procedures required in this resolution. The Executive Committee of the Board is charged with review of all such publications from time to time to ensure that they do not take on the character of formal research reports of the National Bureau, requiring formal Board approval.

7. Unless otherwise determined by the Board or exempted by the terms of paragraph 6, a copy of this resolution shall be printed in each National Bureau publication.

(Resolution adopted October 25, 1926, and revised February 6, 1933,
February 24, 1941, and April 20, 1968)

CONTENTS

TABLES

FOREWORD

The distinction between health and medical care has been a major concern of the National Bureau's health research program ever since its inception some five years ago. Evidence of this concern is apparent in most of the papers published in *Essays in the Economics of Health and Medical Care* and especially in the contribution of Auster, Leveson, and Sarachek, "The Production of Health: An Exploratory Study." The richest and most elegant theoretical treatment of this distinction, however, is in this new study by Michael Grossman. Drawing on some basic notions of Gary Becker's concerning the household's role in the production of ultimate commodities, Grossman has fashioned a model which is theoretically sound, intuitively appealing, and yields significant testable implications.

Prior to Grossman, studies of the demand for medical care were typically set in the framework of consumer demand for a final product and were thought to depend upon prices, income, and "tastes." Tastes were thought to depend in part on state of health, which was exogenously determined. In Grossman's model, people, to some extent, *choose* their level of health just as they choose the level of consumption of other "commodities." Variables such as age and schooling affect demand by altering the "price" of health.

When he turns to the production of health, Grossman realistically assumes that medical care is one input but not the only one. He asks what factors might affect the efficiency of individuals and families in producing health and he presents a substantial amount of evidence indicating that schooling might be one such factor. There are admittedly many possible alternative explanations for the high correlation between health and schooling but Grossman has at least provided one plausible hypothesis within a sensible economic model.

Grossman also shows both theoretically and empirically that higher income does not necessarily lead to higher levels of health, even on average. His explanation is that higher income may also induce higher levels of consumption of other goods and services that have negative effects on health. He has applied the same model to data for individuals and to average data for states and has obtained very similar results. The empirical portion of his work represents a significant advance because of his use of disability and restricted activity as measures of health in addition to the customary one of mortality.

This study, which was awarded the Harry G. Friedman prize by Columbia University for the best dissertation defended in economics in 1970, was supported by grants by the Commonwealth Fund and the National Center for Health Services Research and Development (PHS grant no. 2 P 01 HS 00451–04). The National Bureau's program in health has also been assisted by an Advisory Committee under the chairmanship first of the late Dr. George James and currently Dr. Kurt Deuschle, of the Mount Sinai School of Medicine. Other members of the committee past and present include Gary S. Becker, Morton Bogdonoff, M.D., James Brindle, Norton Brown, M.D., Eveline Burns, Philip E. Enterline, Marion B. Folsom, Eli Ginzberg, William Gorham, Richard Kessler, M.D., the late David Lyall, M.D., Jacob Mincer, Melvin Reder, Peter Rogatz, M.D., James Strickler, M.D., and Gus Tyler.

VICTOR R. FUCHS

ACKNOWLEDGMENTS

This study has been conducted at the National Bureau of Economic Research as part of the economics of health project. My greatest debt is to Gary S. Becker. He suggested the general topic of this study and supervised the work at all stages. When what started out as a relatively simple project developed into a somewhat complex one, his commitment and time input increased. For his help and for the rigorous training in economic theory that he gave me, I am deeply grateful.

I wish to thank many persons at the National Bureau for their help. Victor R. Fuchs made many valuable comments on earlier drafts of this study, encouraged me, particularly when "the going got tough," and tried at all points to transmit his very special research skills to me. Jacob Mincer made several helpful suggestions concerning the empirical implementation of my model and the interpretation of some of the results. Robert T. Michael and Gilbert R. Ghez have done research in areas related to my own and were always willing to discuss difficult theoretical and empirical issues with me. Walter D. Fisher, Kelvin J. Lancaster and W. Allen Wallis read the entire manuscript very thoroughly for the Board of Directors' Reading Committee, and I appreciate their time and effort. Robert Linn and Carol Breckner were extremely able research assistants, and Charlotte Boschan, Susan Crayne, and Martha Jones helped me with computer problems. I am also grateful to Gnomi Schrift Gouldin for editing the manuscript and to H. Irving Forman for drawing the charts.

This study would not have been possible if the Center for Health Administration Studies of the University of Chicago had not been kind enough to make the data from its 1963 health survey available to me. Ronald Anderson supervised the creation of my data decks, and I want to thank him for all his help. I owe a second debt to the Center because I was a member of its research staff during the last year of this project, during which time my research was supported by PHS grant no. HS 00080 from the National Center for Health Services Research and Development.

Finally, I would like to thank my wife Ilene for everything — for drawing diagrams and writing the mathematical formulas in the preliminary drafts and especially for tolerating me while I was working on this project.

INTRODUCTION AND SUMMARY

The aims of this study are to construct and estimate a model of the demand for the commodity "good health." Such a model is important for two reasons. First, the level of ill health, measured by the rates of mortality and morbidity, influences the amount and productivity of labor supplied to an economy. Second, most students of medical economics have long realized that what consumers demand when they purchase medical services are not these services per se but rather "good health."

Early economists related variations in health to starvation. According to the Malthusian theory of population, income fluctuated around a subsistence level. Any temporary increase in income would reduce the rates of mortality and morbidity by improving nutritional and health standards. In modern, developed economies, per capita income far exceeds a subsistence level, at least for a large majority of the population. Therefore, fluctuations in income can no longer be the major determinant of variations in mortality and morbidity. Although in recent years there have been a number of extremely interesting explorations of the forces associated with geographic differences in mortality,[1] these studies have not developed behavioral models that can predict the effects that are in fact observed. For example, why should the age-adjusted mortality rate be *positively* correlated with income across states of the United States, particularly when income and the quantity and quality of medical care are also positively correlated? Again, why should the death rate in the United States be higher than that in many less developed countries? The framework developed in this study can answer these questions and others

[1] See, for example, Irma Adelman, "An Econometric Analysis of Population Growth," *American Economic Review*, 53, No. 3 (June 1963); Richard D. Auster, Irving Leveson, and Deborah Sarachek, "The Production of Health, an Exploratory Study," *Journal of Human Resources*, 4, No. 4 (Fall 1969), and reprinted as Chapter 8 in Victor R. Fuchs (ed.), *Essays in the Economics of Health and Medical Care*, New York, NBER, 1972; Victor R. Fuchs, "Some Economic Aspects of Mortality in the United States," New York, NBER, mimeographed, 1965; Mary Lou Larmore, "An Inquiry into an Econometric Production Function for Health in the United States," unpublished Ph.D. dissertation, Northwestern University, 1967; and Joseph P. Newhouse, "Toward a Rational Allocation of Resources in Medical Care," unpublished Ph.D. dissertation, Harvard University, 1968.

and consequently is one promising way to bridge the existing gap between theory and empiricism in the analysis of health differentials.

Given that the fundamental demand is for good health, it seems logical to study the demand for medical care by first constructing a model of the demand for health itself. Existing models of the demand for health services have not, however, taken this approach. Instead, these models take account of the difference between health and medical care primarily by stressing the importance of variables other than price and income —variables that enter the "taste matrix"—in the demand curve for medical care. For instance, Herbert E. Klarman states that the set of variables in this matrix includes "a person's state of health and his perceptions of and attitudes toward medical care."[2] And Paul J. Feldstein advocates the use of demographic characteristics, like age and education, to measure perceptions and attitudes.[3] Such models of medical care are unsatisfactory because economic analysis does not explain the formation of tastes and thus cannot predict the effects of shifts in taste variables on the demand for health services. It seems quite obvious, for example, that a deterioration in a consumer's health status will cause his medical outlays to increase, but one cannot forecast this effect if health status enters the taste matrix. Again, one may find empirically that the more educated exhibit higher or lower outlays than the less educated, but from models relying on a taste matrix, this finding can only be rationalized in an ad hoc fashion. A complete understanding of the demand for medical care is particularly important because of the rapid increase in its price and share in national income over time. Moreover, government programs play a key role in the medical sector. To maximize the effectiveness of these programs, policy makers must be able to predict the impact of shifts in a wide number of variables on the demand for health and medical care.

Since traditional demand theory assumes that goods and services purchased in the market enter consumers' utility functions, it is obvious why economists have emphasized the demand for medical care at the expense of the demand for health. Fortunately, a new approach to consumer behavior draws a sharp distinction between fundamental objects of choice—called commodities—and market goods.[4] Thus, it

[2] *The Economics of Health*, New York, 1965, p. 25.

[3] "Research on the Demand for Health Services," *Milbank Memorial Fund Quarterly*, 44, No. 4, Part 2 (October 1966), p. 143.

[4] See Gary S. Becker, "A Theory of the Allocation of Time," *Economic Journal*, 75, No. 299 (September 1965); Gary S. Becker and Robert T. Michael, "On the Theory of Consumer Demand," unpublished paper, 1970; Kelvin J. Lancaster, "A New Approach to Consumer Theory," *Journal of Political Economy*, 75, No. 2 (April 1966); and Richard Muth, "Household Production and Consumer Demand Functions," *Econometrica*, 34, No. 3 (July 1966).

serves as the point of departure for the health model utilized in this study. In this approach, consumers *produce* commodities with inputs of market goods and their own time. For example, they use sporting equipment and their own time to produce recreation, traveling time and transportation services to produce visits, and part of their Sundays and church services to produce "peace of mind." Since goods and services are inputs into the production of commodities, the demand for these goods and services is a derived demand.

Within the new framework for examining consumer behavior, the commodity good health is treated as a durable item. This treatment is adopted because "health capital" is one component of human capital, and the latter has been treated as a stock in the literature on investment in human beings.[5] Consequently, it is assumed that individuals inherit an initial stock of health that depreciates over time—at an increasing rate, at least after some stage in the life cycle—and can be increased by investment. Direct inputs into the production of gross investments in the stock of health include own time, medical care, diet, exercise, housing, and other market goods as well. The production function also depends on certain "environmental variables," the most important of which is the level of education of the producer, that alter the efficiency of the production process.

It should be realized that in this model the level of health of an individual is *not* exogenous but depends, at least in part, on the resources allocated to its production. Health is demanded by consumers for two reasons. As a consumption commodity, it directly enters their preference functions, or put differently, sick days are a source of disutility. As an investment commodity, it determines the total amount of time available for market and nonmarket activities. In other words, an increase in the stock of health reduces the time lost from these activities, and the monetary value of this reduction is an index of the return to an investment in health.

Since the most fundamental law in economics is the law of the downward sloping demand curve, the quantity of health demanded should be negatively correlated with its *shadow price*. The analysis in the theoretical sections of this study stresses that the shadow price of health depends on many variables besides the price of medical care. Shifts in these variables alter the optimal amount of health and also the derived demand for gross investment (measured, say, by medical expenditures).

[5] See, for example, Gary S. Becker, *Human Capital and the Personal Distribution of Income: An Analytical Approach*, W. S. Woytinsky Lecture No. 1, Ann Arbor, Michigan, 1967; and Yoram Ben-Porath, "The Production of Human Capital and the Life Cycle of Earnings," *Journal of Political Economy*, 75, No. 4 (August 1967).

It is shown that the shadow price rises with age if the rate of depreciation on the stock of health rises over the life cycle, and falls with education if more educated people are more efficient producers of health. This price may also be related to wealth, wage rates, and other variables as well. Of particular importance is the conclusion that, under certain conditions, an increase in the shadow price may simultaneously reduce the quantity of health demanded and increase the quantity of medical care demanded.

The empirical sections of the study estimate demand curves for health and medical care and gross investment production functions. The demand curves are fitted by ordinary least squares and the production functions by two-stage least squares. The principal data source is the 1963 health interview survey conducted by the National Opinion Research Center and the Center for Health Administration Studies of the University of Chicago. Health capital is measured by individuals' self-evaluation of their health status. Healthy time, the output produced by health capital, is measured either by the complement of the number of restricted-activity days due to illness and injury or by the complement of the number of work-loss days. The main independent variables in the health and medical care regressions are the age of the individual, the number of years of formal schooling he or she completed, his or her weekly wage rate, and family income.

The most important regression results are as follows. Education has a positive and statistically significant coefficient in the health demand curve. The marginal cost of producing gross additions to health capital is roughly 7.1 percent lower for consumers with, say, eleven years of formal schooling compared to those with ten years. An increase in age simultaneously reduces health and increases medical expenditures. Computations based on the age coefficients reveal that the continuously compounded rate of growth of the depreciation rate is 2.1 percent per year over the life cycle. The best estimate of the price elasticity of demand for health is .5. Estimates of the elasticity of health with respect to medical care range from .1 to .3. The wage elasticity of health is positive and statistically significant.

The most surprising finding is that healthy time has a negative income elasticity. If the consumption aspects of health were at all relevant, then a literal interpretation of the observed income effect would suggest that health is an inferior commodity; however, this is not the only possible interpretation of the results. The explanation offered in the study stresses that medical care is not the only market input in the gross investment production function. Instead, inputs such as housing, recreation goods, alcohol, cigarettes, and rich food are also relevant. The last three inputs have negative marginal products, and if their income elasticities exceeded the income elasticities of the beneficial inputs, the marginal cost of gross investment would be positively correlated with income. This appears to be a promising explanation because it can also account for the observed positive income elasticity of medical care. That is, it can show the conditions under which higher income persons would simultaneously reduce their demand for health and increase their demand for medical care.

The empirical analysis also assesses the impact of disability insurance —insurance that finances earnings lost due to illness—on work-loss. Moreover, to check the results obtained when ill health is measured by sick time, variations in death rates across states of the United States are studied. This analysis reveals a remarkable qualitative and quantitative agreement between the mortality and sick time regression coefficients. Although not all its theoretical predictions are fulfilled, enough are to suggest that the model developed here provides a viable framework for understanding variations in health levels and medical expenditures.

THE DEMAND FOR HEALTH:
A THEORETICAL AND EMPIRICAL
INVESTIGATION

I

A STOCK APPROACH TO THE DEMAND FOR HEALTH

In this chapter, I develop a model to analyze the demand for the commodity good health. The central proposition of the model is that health is a durable commodity. Individuals are said to inherit an initial stock of health that depreciates over time and can be augmented by investment. Death is said to occur when the stock falls below a certain level, and one of the novel features of the model is that individuals "choose" their length of life. I first describe how a given consumer selects the optimal amount of health in any period of his life. I then formalize the equilibrium conditions for health and the other arguments of the utility function and also comment on some general features of the model.

1. THE MODEL

Let the intertemporal utility function of a typical consumer be

$$U = U(\phi_0 H_0, \ldots, \phi_n H_n, Z_0, \ldots, Z_n), \qquad (1\text{-}1)$$

where H_0 is the inherited stock of health, H_i is the stock of health in the ith time period, ϕ_i is the service flow per unit stock, $h_i = \phi_i H_i$ is total consumption of "health services," and Z_i is total consumption of another commodity[1] in the ith period.[2] Note that whereas in the usual intertemporal utility function, the length of life (n) as of the planning date is fixed, here it is an endogenous variable. In particular, death takes place when $H_i = H_{\min}$. Therefore, length of life depends on the quantities of H_i that maximize utility subject to certain production and resource constraints that are now outlined.

By definition, net investment in the stock of health equals gross investment minus depreciation:

$$H_{i+1} - H_i = I_i - \delta_i H_i, \qquad (1\text{-}2)$$

where I_i is gross investment and δ_i is the rate of depreciation during the ith period. The rates of depreciation are assumed to be exogenous, but

---

[1] The commodity Z_i may be viewed as an aggregate of all commodities besides health that enter the utility function in period i.

[2] For the convenience of the reader, a glossary of symbols follows each chapter.

they may vary with the age of the individual.[3] Consumers produce gross investments in health and the other commodities in the utility function according to a set of household production functions:

$$I_i = I_i(M_i, TH_i; E_i)$$
$$Z_i = Z_i(X_i, T_i; E_i).$$
(1-3)

In these equations, M_i is medical care, X_i is the goods input in the production of the commodity Z_i, T_i and TH_i are time inputs, and E_i is the stock of human capital.[4] It is assumed that a shift in human capital changes the efficiency of the production process in the nonmarket sector of the economy, just as a shift in technology changes the efficiency of the production process in the market sector. The implications of this treatment of human capital are explored in Chapter II.

It is also assumed that all production functions are homogeneous of degree one in the goods and time inputs. Therefore, the gross investment production can be written as

$$I_i = M_i g(t_i; E_i),$$
(1-4)

where $t_i = TH_i/M_i$. It follows that the marginal products of time and medical care in the production of gross investment in health are

$$\frac{\partial I_i}{\partial TH_i} = \frac{\partial g}{\partial t_i} = g'$$
$$\frac{\partial I_i}{\partial M_i} = g - t_i g'.$$
(1-5)

From the point of view of the individual, both market goods and own time are scarce resources. The goods budget constraint equates the

[3] In a more complicated version of the model, the rate of depreciation might be a negative function of the stock of health. The analysis is considerably simplified by treating this rate as exogenous, and the conclusions reached would tend to hold even if it were endogenous.

[4] In general, medical care is not the only market good in the gross investment function, for inputs such as housing, diet, recreation, cigarette smoking, and alcohol consumption influence one's level of health. Since these inputs also produce other commodities in the utility function, joint production occurs in the household. For an analysis of this phenomenon, see Chapter VI. Until then, medical care is treated as the most important market good in the gross investment function. This treatment is adopted because the other inputs are difficult to measure empirically.

present value of outlays on goods to the present value of earnings income over the life cycle plus initial assets (discounted property income):[5]

$$\sum \frac{P_i M_i + F_i X_i}{(1 + r)^i} = \sum \frac{W_i T W_i}{(1 + r)^i} + A_0. \tag{1-6}$$

Here P_i and F_i are the prices of M_i and X_i, W_i is the wage rate, TW_i is hours of work, A_0 is discounted property income, and r is the interest rate. The time constraint requires that Ω, the total amount of time available in any period, must be exhausted by all possible uses:

$$TW_i + TH_i + T_i + TL_i = \Omega, \tag{1-7}$$

where TL_i is time lost from market and nonmarket activities due to illness or injury.

Equation (1-7) modifies the time budget constraint in Gary S. Becker's time model.[6] If sick time were not added to market and non-market time, total time would *not* be exhausted by all possible uses. My model assumes that TL_i is inversely related to the stock of health; that is, $\partial TL_i / \partial H_i < 0$. If Ω were measured in days ($\Omega = 365$ days if a year is the relevant period) and if ϕ_i were defined as the flow of healthy days yielded by a unit of H_i, h_i would equal the total number of healthy days in a given year.[7] Then one could write

$$TL_i = \Omega - h_i. \tag{1-8}$$

It is important to draw a sharp distinction between sick time and the time input in the gross investment function. As an illustration of this difference, the time a consumer allocates to visiting his doctor for periodic checkups is obviously not sick time. More formally, if the rate of depreciation were held constant, an increase in TH_i would increase I_i and H_{i+1} and would reduce TL_{i+1}. Thus, TH_i and TL_{i+1} would be negatively correlated.[8]

By substituting for TW_i from equation (1-7) into equation (1-6), one obtains the single "full wealth" constraint

$$\sum \frac{P_i M_i + F_i X_i + W_i(TH_i + T_i + TL_i)}{(1 + r)^i} = \sum \frac{W_i \Omega}{(1 + r)^i} + A_0 = R. \tag{1-9}$$

[5] Except where indicated, the sums throughout this study are taken from $i = 0$ to n.

[6] See "A Theory of the Allocation of Time," *Economic Journal*, 75, No. 299 (September 1965).

[7] If the stock of health yielded other services besides healthy days, ϕ_i would be a vector of service flows. This study emphasizes the service flow of healthy days because this flow can be measured empirically.

[8] For a discussion of conditions that would produce a positive correlation between TH_i and TL_{i+1}, see Chapter II, Section 2.

According to equation (1-9), full wealth equals initial assets plus the present value of the earnings an individual would obtain if he spent all of his time at work. Part of this wealth is spent on market goods, part of it is spent on nonmarket production time, and part of it is lost due to illness. The equilibrium quantities of H_i and Z_i can now be found by maximizing the utility function given by equation (1-1) subject to the constraints given by equations (1-2), (1-3), and (1-9).[9] Since the inherited stock of health and the rates of depreciation are given, the optimal quantities of gross investment determine the optimal quantities of health capital.

2. EQUILIBRIUM CONDITIONS

First order optimality conditions for gross investment in period $i - 1$ are[10]

$$\frac{\pi_{i-1}}{(1+r)^{i-1}} = \frac{W_i G_i}{(1+r)^i} + \frac{(1-\delta_i)W_{i+1}G_{i+1}}{(1+r)^{i+1}} + \cdots$$

$$+ \frac{(1-\delta_i)\ldots(1-\delta_{n-1})W_n G_n}{(1+r)^n}$$

$$+ \frac{Uh_i G_i}{\lambda} + \cdots + (1-\delta_i)\ldots(1-\delta_{n-1})\frac{Uh_n G_n}{\lambda}. \qquad (1\text{-}10)$$

$$\pi_{i-1} = \frac{P_{i-1}}{g - t_{i-1}g'} = \frac{W_{i-1}}{g'}. \qquad (1\text{-}11)$$

The new symbols in these equations are Uh_i, the marginal utility of healthy days; λ, the marginal utility of wealth; $G_i = \partial h_i/\partial H_i = -\partial TL/\partial H_i$, the marginal product of the stock of health in the production of healthy days; π_{i-1}, the marginal cost of gross investment in health in period $i - 1$.

Equation (1-10) simply states that the present value of the marginal cost of gross investment in period $i - 1$ must equal the present value

---

[9] In addition, the constraint is imposed that $H_n \leq H_{\min}$.

[10] Note that an increase in gross investment in period $i - 1$ increases the stock of health in all future periods. These increases are equal to $\partial H_i/\partial I_{i-1} = 1$, $\partial H_{i+1}/\partial I_{i-1} = (1-\delta_i), \ldots,$ $\partial H_n/\partial I_{i-1} = (1-\delta_i)(1-\delta_{i+1})\ldots(1-\delta_{n-1})$. Note also that if Z_i were nondurable, its first order conditions would be

$$\frac{U_i}{\lambda} = \frac{q_i}{(1+r)^i}, \qquad q_i = \frac{F_i}{\partial Z_i/\partial X_i} = \frac{W_i}{\partial Z_i/\partial T_i}.$$

For a derivation of equation (1-10), see Appendix A, Section 1.

of marginal benefits. Discounted marginal benefits at age i equal $G_i[W_i(1 + r)^{-i} + Uh_i\lambda^{-1}]$, where G_i is the marginal product of health capital—the increase in the number of healthy days caused by a one unit increase in the stock of health. Two monetary magnitudes are necessary to convert this marginal product into value terms because consumers desire health for two reasons. The discounted wage rate measures the monetary value of a one unit increase in the total amount of time available for market and nonmarket activities, and the term Uh_i/λ measures the discounted monetary equivalent of the increase in utility due to a one unit increase in healthy time. Thus, the sum of these two terms measures the discounted marginal value to consumers of the output produced by health capital.

While equation (1-10) determines the optimal amount of gross investment in period $i - 1$, equation (1-11) shows the condition for minimizing the cost of producing a given quantity of gross investment. Total cost is minimized when the change in gross investment from spending an additional dollar on medical care equals the change in gross investment from spending an additional dollar on time. Since the gross investment production function is homogeneous of degree one and since the prices of medical care and own time are independent of the level of these inputs, average cost is constant and equal to marginal cost.

To examine the forces that affect the demand for health and gross investment, it is useful to convert equation (1-10) into a slightly different form. If gross investment in period i is positive, then:

$$\frac{\pi_i}{(1 + r)^i} = \frac{W_{i+1}G_{i+1}}{(1 + r)^{i+1}} + \frac{(1 - \delta_{i+1})W_{i+2}G_{i+2}}{(1 + r)^{i+2}} + \cdots$$

$$+ \frac{(1 - \delta_{i+1})\ldots(1 - \delta_{n-1})W_nG_n}{(1 + r)^n} + \frac{Uh_{i+1}}{\lambda}G_{i+1} + \cdots$$

$$+ (1 - \delta_{i+1})\ldots(1 - \delta_{n-1})\frac{Uh_n}{\lambda}G_n. \tag{1-12}$$

From (1-10) and (1-12),

$$\frac{\pi_{i-1}}{(1 + r)^{i-1}} = \frac{W_iG_i}{(1 + r)^i} + \frac{Uh_i}{\lambda}G_i + \frac{(1 - \delta_i)\pi_i}{(1 + r)^i}.$$

Therefore,

$$G_i[W_i + (Uh_i/\lambda)(1 + r)^i] = \pi_{i-1}(r - \tilde{\pi}_{i-1} + \delta_i), \tag{1-13}$$

where $\tilde{\pi}_{i-1}$ is the percentage rate of change in marginal cost between period $i-1$ and period i.[11] Equation (1-13) implies that the undiscounted value of the marginal product of the optimal stock of health capital at any moment in time must equal the supply price of capital, $\pi_{i-1}(r - \tilde{\pi}_{i-1} + \delta_i)$. The latter contains interest, depreciation, and capital gains components and may be interpreted as the rental price or user cost of health capital.

Condition (1-13) fully determines the demand for capital goods that can be bought and sold in a perfect market. In such a market, if firms or households acquire one unit of stock in period $i-1$ at price π_{i-1}, they can sell $(1 - \delta_i)$ units at price π_i at the end of period i. Consequently, $\pi_{i-1}(r - \tilde{\pi}_{i-1} + \delta_i)$ measures the cost of holding one unit of capital for one period. The transaction just described allows individuals to raise their capital in period i *alone* by one unit and is clearly feasible for stocks like automobiles, houses, refrigerators, and producer durables. It suggests that one can define a set of single period flow equilibria for stocks that last for many periods.

In my model, the stock of health capital cannot be sold in the capital market, just as the stock of knowledge cannot be sold. This means that gross investment must be nonnegative. Although sales of health capital are ruled out, provided gross investment is positive, there exists a user cost of capital that in equilibrium must equal the value of the marginal product of the stock.[12] An intuitive interpretation of this result is that exchanges over time in the stock of health by an individual substitute for exchanges in the capital market. Suppose a consumer desires to increase his stock of health by one unit in period i. Then he must increase gross investment in period $i-1$ by one unit. If he simultaneously reduces gross investment in period i by $(1 - \delta_i)$ units, then he has engaged in a transaction that raises H_i, and H_i *alone*, by one unit. Put differently, he has essentially rented one unit of capital from himself for one period. The magnitude of the reduction in I_i is smaller the greater the rate of depreciation, and its dollar value is larger the greater the rate of increase in marginal cost over time. Thus, the depreciation and capital gains components are as relevant to the user cost of health as they are to the user cost of any other durable. Of course, the interest component of user cost is easy to interpret, for if one desires to increase his stock of health rather

---

[11] Equation (1-13) assumes $\delta_i \tilde{\pi}_{i-1} \simeq 0$.

[12] For a similar conclusion, see Kenneth J. Arrow, "Optimal Capital Policy with Irreversible Investment," in J. N. Wolfe (ed.), *Value, Capital and Growth: Papers in Honour of Sir John Hicks*, Edinburgh, 1968.

than his stock of some other asset by one unit in a given period, $r\pi_{i-1}$ measures the interest payment he foregoes.[13]

A slightly different form of equation (1-13) emerges if both sides are divided by the marginal cost of gross investment:

$$\gamma_i + a_i = r - \tilde{\pi}_{i-1} + \delta_i. \tag{1-13'}$$

Here $\gamma_i = W_i G_i / \pi_{i-1}$ is the marginal monetary rate of return to an investment in health and $a_i = [(U h_i / \lambda)(1 + r)^i G_i] / \pi_{i-1}$ is the psychic rate of return. In equilibrium, the total rate of return to an investment in health must equal the user cost of health capital in terms of the price of gross investment. The latter variable is defined as the sum of the real-own rate of interest and the rate of depreciation.

In Chapters II and III, equation (1-13') is used to trace out the lifetime path of health and gross investment, to explore the effects of variations in depreciation rates, and to examine the impact of changes in the marginal cost of gross investment. Before turning our attention to these matters, let us consider the following general properties of the model. It should be realized that equation (1-13') breaks down whenever desired gross investment equals zero. In this situation, the present value of the marginal cost of gross investment would exceed the present value of marginal benefits for all positive quantities of gross investment, and equations (1-10) and (1-12) would be replaced by inequalities.[14] The discussion in the remainder of this study rules out zero gross investment by assumption, but the conclusions reached would have to be modified if this were not the case.

It should also be realized that since there are constant returns to scale in the production of gross investment and since input prices are given, the marginal cost of gross investment and its percentage rate of change over time are exogenous variables. Put differently, these two variables are independent of the rate of investment and the stock of health. This implies that consumers reach their desired stock of capital immediately. It also implies that the stock rather than gross investment is the basic decision variable in the model. By this I mean that consumers respond to changes in the cost of capital by altering the marginal product

[13] In a continuous time model, the user cost of health capital can be derived in one step. If continuous time is employed, the term $\delta_i \tilde{\pi}_{i-1}$ does not appear in the user cost formula. The right-hand side of (1-13) becomes $\pi_i(r - \tilde{\pi}_i + \delta_i)$, where $\tilde{\pi}_i$ is the instantaneous percentage rate of change of marginal cost at age i. For a proof, see Appendix A, Section 2.

[14] Formally, $\gamma_i + a_i \leq r - \tilde{\pi}_{i-1} + \delta_i$, if $I_{i-1} = I_i = 0$.

of health capital and not the marginal cost of gross investment.[15] Therefore, even though equation (1-13′) is not independent of equations (1-10)
and (1-12), it can be used to determine the optimal path of health capital
and by implication the optimal path of gross investment.[16]

It is clear that the number of sick days and the number of healthy
days are complements; their sum equals the constant length of the period.
From equation (1-8) the marginal utility of sick time is $-Uh_i$. Thus, by
putting healthy days in the utility function, one implicitly assumes that
sick days yield *disutility*. If healthy days did not enter the utility function
directly, the monetary rate of return would equal the cost of health
capital, and health would be solely an investment commodity.[17]

The monetary returns to an investment in health differ from the
returns to investments in education, on-the-job training, and other forms
of human capital since the latter investments raise wage rates.[18] Of course,
the amount of health capital might influence the wage rate, but it necessarily influences the time lost from all activities due to illness or injury.
To emphasize the novelty of my approach, I assume that health is not a
determinant of the wage rate. Put differently, a person's stock of knowledge affects his market and nonmarket productivity, while his stock of
health determines the total amount of time he can spend producing
money earnings and commodities.[19] Since both market and nonmarket
time are relevant, even individuals who are not in the labor force have an
incentive to invest in their health. For such individuals, the marginal
product of health capital would be converted into a dollar equivalent by
multiplying by the monetary value of the marginal utility of time.

I have been reluctant to label health either pure consumption
($\gamma_i = 0$) or pure investment ($Uh_i = 0$) because many observers believe

[15] In Chapter II, it is shown that if the marginal disutility of sick time equals zero, the
determination of the equilibrium stock of capital in period i requires diminishing marginal
productivity of capital. For a model in which gross investment is the basic decision variable,
see Yoram Ben-Porath, "The Production of Human Capital and the Life Cycle of Earnings,"
Journal of Political Economy, 75, No. 4 (August 1967). Ben-Porath assumes that the marginal
product of the stock of knowledge is constant, but the marginal cost of producing gross
additions to the stock is positively related to the rate of gross investment.

[16] This statement is subject to the modification that the optimal path of capital must
always imply nonnegative gross investment.

[17] To avoid confusion, a note on terminology is in order. If health were entirely an
investment commodity, it would yield monetary, but not utility, returns. Regardless of whether
health is investment, consumption, or a mixture of the two, one can speak of a *gross investment
function* since the commodity in question is a durable.

[18] This difference is emphasized by Selma J. Mushkin in "Health as an Investment,"
Journal of Political Economy, 70, No. 5, Part 2 (October 1962), pp. 132–133.

[19] Hence, E_i, the stock of knowledge or human capital, does *not* include health capital.

the demand for it has both investment and consumption aspects.[20] But to simplify the theoretical analysis, Chapter II offers a pure investment interpretation of a certain set of phenomena, while Chapter III offers a pure consumption interpretation of the same set. In both frameworks, the assumption of constant marginal cost guarantees instantaneous adjustments to variables that shift the demand for health in a once and for all fashion. Therefore, there would be no net investment or disinvestment over the life cycle of an individual unless his demand for health were a function of time.

3. GLOSSARY

n	Total length of life
i	Age
H_0	Inherited stock of health
H_i	Stock of health in period i
H_{min}	Death stock
ψ_i	Service flow per unit stock or number of healthy days per unit stock
h_i	Total number of healthy days in period i
Z_i	Consumption of an aggregate commodity in period i
I_i	Gross investment in health
δ_i	Rate of depreciation
M_i	Medical care
TH_i	Time input in gross investment function
X_i	Goods input in the production of Z_i
T_i	Time input in the production of Z_i
E_i	Stock of human capital
$g - t_i g'$	Marginal product of medical care in the gross investment production function
g'	Marginal product of time
P_i	Price of medical care
F_i	Price of X_i
W_i	Wage rate
A_0	Initial assets
r	Rate of interest

[20] See, for example, Mushkin, *op. cit.*, p. 131; and Victor R. Fuchs, "The Contribution of Health Services to the American Economy," *Milbank Memorial Fund Quarterly*, 44, No. 4, Part 2 (October 1966), p. 86, and reprinted as Chapter 1 in *Essays in the Economics of Health and Medical Care*, New York, NBER, 1972.

TW_i	Hours of work
TL_i	Sick time
Ω	Constant length of the period
R	Full wealth
G_i	Marginal product of health capital
Uh_i	Marginal utility of healthy days
λ	Marginal utility of wealth
π_i	Marginal cost of gross investment in health
$\tilde{\pi}_i$	Percentage rate of change in marginal cost
q_i	Marginal cost of Z_i
γ_i	Monetary rate of return on an investment in health or marginal efficiency of health capital
a_i	Psychic rate of return on an investment in health

II

THE SHADOW PRICE OF HEALTH

In the previous chapter, I showed how a consumer selects the optimal quantity of health in any period of his life. In this chapter, I explore the effects of changes in the supply and demand prices of health in the context of the pure investment model. In Section 1, I comment on the demand curve for health capital in the investment model. In Section 2, I relate variations in depreciation rates with age to life cycle patterns of health and gross investment. I also examine the impact of changes in depreciation rates among individuals of the same age and briefly incorporate uncertainty into the model. In the third section, I consider the effects of shifts in market efficiency, measured by the wage rate, and nonmarket efficiency, measured by human capital, on supply and demand prices.

1. THE INVESTMENT DEMAND CURVE

If the marginal utility of healthy days or the marginal disutility of sick days were equal to zero, health would be solely an investment commodity. The optimal amount of H_i could then be found by equating the marginal monetary rate of return on an investment in health to the cost of health capital:

$$W_i G_i / \pi_{i-1} = \gamma_i = r - \tilde{\pi}_{i-1} + \delta_i. \tag{2-1}$$

Setting $Uh_i = 0$ in equation (1-13'), one derives equation (2-1). It can also be derived by excluding health from the utility function and redefining the full wealth constraint as

$$R' = A_0 + \sum \frac{W_i h_i - \pi_i I_i}{(1 + r)^i} \tag{2-2}$$

Maximization of R' with respect to gross investment in periods $i - 1$ and i yields condition (2-1).[1]

---

[1] For a proof, see Appendix B, Section 1. The continuous time version of (2-1) is

$$W_i G_i / \pi_i = \gamma_i = r - \tilde{\pi}_i + \delta_i,$$

where $\tilde{\pi}_i$ is the instantaneous percentage rate of change in marginal cost. This equation, too, is derived in Appendix B, Section 1.

Figure 1 illustrates the determination of the optimal stock of health capital at any age i. The demand curve MEC shows the relationship between the stock of health and the rate of return on an investment or the marginal efficiency of health capital. The supply curve S shows the relationship between the stock of health and the cost of capital. Since the real-own rate of interest and the rate of depreciation are independent of the stock, the supply curve is infinitely elastic. Provided the MEC schedule slopes downward, the equilibrium stock is given by H_i^*, where the supply and demand curves intersect.

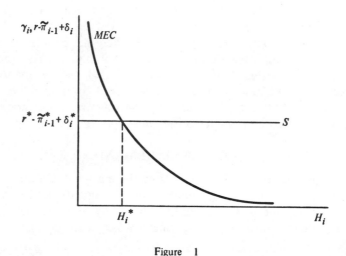

Figure   1

In the model, the wage rate and the marginal cost of gross investment do not depend on the stock of health. Therefore, the MEC schedule would be negatively inclined if and only if the marginal product of health capital were diminishing. Since the output produced by health capital has a finite upper limit of 365 healthy days, it seems reasonable to assume diminishing marginal productivity. Figure 2 shows a plausible relationship between the stock of health and the number of healthy days. This relationship may be called the production function of healthy days. The slope of the curve in the figure at any point gives the marginal product of health capital. The number of healthy days equals zero at the death stock, H_{min}, so that $\Omega = TL_i = 365$ is an alternative definition of death. Beyond H_{min}, healthy time increases at a decreasing rate and eventually

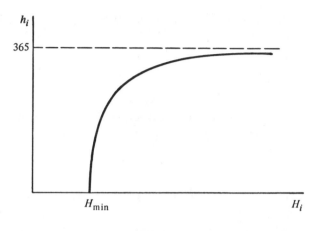

Figure   2

approaches its upper asymptote of 365 days as the stock becomes large.[2]

2. VARIATIONS IN DEPRECIATION RATES

Life Cycle Patterns

Equation (2-1) enables one to study the behavior of the demand for health and gross investment over the life cycle. To simplify the analysis, it is assumed that the wage rate, the stock of knowledge, the marginal cost of gross investment, and the marginal productivity of health capital are independent of age. These assumptions are not as restrictive as they may seem. To be sure, wage rates and human capital are undoubtedly correlated with age, but the effects of shifts in these variables are treated in Section 3. Therefore, the results obtained in this section may be viewed as *partial* effects. That is, they show the impact of a *pure* increase in age on the demand for health, with all other variables held constant.[3]

[2] Certain production functions might exhibit upper asymptotes but increasing or constant marginal productivity in some regions. In general, if discontinuities in the MEC schedule are ruled out, the sufficient condition for maximizing R' with respect to H_i requires diminishing marginal productivity in the vicinity of the equilibrium stock. For a complete discussion of this point, see Appendix B, Section 1.

[3] For an analysis of life cycle phenomena that allows wage rates and human capital to vary with age, see equation (2-21).

Since marginal cost does not depend on age, $\tilde{\pi}_{i-1} = 0$, and equation (2-1) reduces to

$$\gamma_i = r + \delta_i. \tag{2-3}$$

It is apparent from equation (2-3) that if the rate of depreciation were independent of age, a single quantity of H would satisfy the equality between the marginal rate of return and the cost of health capital. Consequently, there would be no net investment or disinvestment after the initial period. One could not, in general, compare H_0 and H_1 because accumulation in the initial period would depend on the discrepancy between the inherited stock and the stock desired in period 1. This discrepancy in turn would be related to variations in H_0 and other variables across individuals. But, given zero costs of adjusting to the desired level immediately, H would be constant after period 1. Under the stated condition of a constant depreciation rate, individuals would choose an infinite life if they choose to live beyond period 1. In other words, if $H_1 > H_{min}$, H_i would always exceed the death stock.[4]

To permit the demand for health to vary with age, assume that the rate of depreciation depends on age. In general, any time path of δ_i is possible. For example, the rate of depreciation might be negatively correlated with age during early stages of the life cycle. Or the time path might be nonmonotonic, so that δ_i rises during some periods and falls during others. Despite the existence of a wide variety of possible time paths, it is extremely plausible to assume that δ_i is positively correlated with age after some point in the life cycle. This correlation can be inferred because as an individual ages, his physical strength and memory capacity deteriorate. Surely, a rise in the rate of depreciation on his stock of health is merely one manifestation of the biological process of aging. Therefore, the analysis focuses on the effects of an increase in the rate of depreciation with age.

Since a rise in δ_i increases the cost of health capital, it would cause the demand for health to fall over the life cycle. Graphically, an upward shift in the cost of capital from $r + \delta_i$ to $r + \delta_{i+1}$ in Figure 3 reduces the optimal stock from H_i to H_{i+1}. The greater is the elasticity of the MEC schedule, the greater the decrease in the optimal stock with age. Put differently, the slower is the increase in the marginal product of health capital as H falls, the greater the decrease in the optimal stock.

---

[4] The possibility that death can occur in period 1 is ruled out from now on.

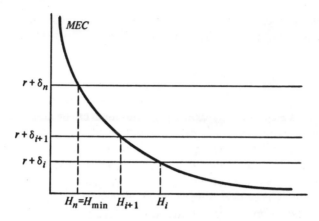

Figure 3

Differentiation of equation (2-3) with respect to age quantifies the percentage rate of decrease in the stock of health over the life cycle:

$$\tilde{H}_i = -s_i \varepsilon_i \tilde{\delta}_i. \tag{2-4}$$

A tilde denotes a percentage time derivative

$$\left(\tilde{H}_i = \frac{dH_i}{di} \frac{1}{H_i}, \text{etc.} \right),$$

where:

$$s_i = \frac{\delta_i}{r + \delta_i} = \text{the share of depreciation in the cost of health capital}$$

$$\varepsilon_i = -\frac{\partial \ln H_i}{\partial \ln (r + \delta_i)} = -\frac{\partial \ln H_i}{\partial \ln \gamma_i} = -\frac{\partial \ln H_i}{\partial \ln G_i}$$

= elasticity of MEC schedule.[5]

Equation (2-4) indicates that the absolute value of the percentage decrease in H is positively related to the elasticity of the MEC schedule, the share of depreciation in the cost of health capital, and the percentage rate of

[5] From equation (2-3), $\ln (r + \delta_i) = \ln W + \ln G_i - \ln \pi$. Therefore,

$$\frac{\delta_i \tilde{\delta}_i}{r + \delta_i} = \frac{\partial \ln G_i}{\partial \ln H_i} \tilde{H}_i, \quad \text{or} \quad s_i \tilde{\delta}_i = -\frac{\tilde{H}_i}{\varepsilon_i}.$$

increase in the rate of depreciation. If ε_i and $\tilde{\delta}_i$ were constant, the curve relating $\ln H_i$ to age would be concave unless $r = 0$ since[6]

$$\frac{d\tilde{H}_i}{di} = \tilde{H}_{ii} = -s_i(1 - s_i)\varepsilon\tilde{\delta}^2 < 0. \tag{2-5}$$

The absolute value of $\tilde{H}_i$ increases over the life cycle because the share of depreciation in the cost of capital rises with age. ·

If δ_i grows continuously with age after some point in the life cycle, persons would choose to live a finite life. Since H declines over the life cycle, it would eventually fall to H_{min}, the death stock. When the cost of health capital is $r + \delta_n$ in Figure 3, $H_n = H_{min}$, and death occurs. At death, no time is available for market and nonmarket activities since healthy time equals zero. Therefore, the monetary equivalent of sick time in period n would completely exhaust potential full earnings, $W\Omega$. Moreover, consumption of the commodity Z_n would equal zero since no time would be available for its production if total time equals sick time.[7] Because individuals could not produce commodities, total utility would be driven to zero at death.[8]

Having characterized the optimal path of H_i, one can proceed to examine the behavior of gross investment. Gross investment's life cycle profile would not, in general, simply mirror that of health capital. In other words, even though health capital falls over the life cycle, gross investment might increase, remain constant, or decrease. This follows because a rise in the rate of depreciation not only reduces the amount of health capital *demanded* by consumers but also reduces the amount of capital *supplied* to them by a given amount of gross investment. If the change in supply exceeded the change in demand, individuals would have an incentive to close this gap by increasing gross investment. On the other hand, if the change in supply were less than the change in demand, gross investment would tend to fall over the life cycle.

---

[6] Differentiation of (2-4) with respect to age yields

$$\tilde{H}_{ii} = -\frac{\varepsilon\tilde{\delta}[(r + \delta_i)\delta_i\tilde{\delta} - \delta_i(\delta_i\tilde{\delta})]}{(r + \delta_i)^2}, \quad \text{or} \quad \tilde{H}_{ii} = -\frac{\delta_i r\varepsilon\tilde{\delta}^2}{(r + \delta_i)^2} = -s_i(1 - s_i)\varepsilon\tilde{\delta}^2.$$

[7] This assumes that Z_i cannot be produced with X_i alone; which would be true if, say, the production function were Cobb-Douglas.

[8] Utility equals zero when $H = H_{min}$ provided the death time utility function is such that $U(0) = 0$.

To predict the effect of an increase in δ_i with age on gross investment, note that net investment can be approximated by $H_i \tilde{H}_i$.[9] Since gross investment equals net investment plus depreciation,

$$\ln I_i = \ln H_i + \ln (\tilde{H}_i + \delta_i). \tag{2-6}$$

Differentiation of equation (2-6) with respect to age yields

$$\tilde{I}_i = \frac{\tilde{H}_i^2 + \delta_i \tilde{H}_i + \tilde{H}_{ii} + \delta_i \tilde{\delta}_i}{\tilde{H}_i + \delta_i}.$$

Suppose $\tilde{\delta}_i$ and ε_i were constant. Then from (2-4) and (2-5), the expression for $\tilde{I}_i$ would simplify to

$$\tilde{I}_i = \frac{\tilde{\delta}(1 - s_i \varepsilon_i)(\delta_i - s_i \varepsilon \tilde{\delta}) + s_i^2 \varepsilon \tilde{\delta}^2}{\delta_i - s_i \varepsilon \tilde{\delta}}. \tag{2-7}$$

Since health capital cannot be sold, gross investment cannot be negative. Therefore, $\delta_i \geq -\tilde{H}_i$.[10] That is, if the stock of health falls over the life cycle, the absolute value of the percentage rate of net disinvestment cannot exceed the rate of depreciation. Provided gross investment does not equal zero, the term $\delta_i - s_i \varepsilon \tilde{\delta}$ in equation (2-7) must exceed zero. It follows that a sufficient condition for gross investment to be positively correlated with the depreciation rate is $\varepsilon < 1/s_i$. Thus, $\tilde{I}_i$ would definitely be positive at every point if $\varepsilon < 1$.

The important conclusion is reached that if the elasticity of the MEC schedule were less than one, gross investment and the depreciation rate would be positively correlated over the life cycle, while gross investment and the stock of health would be negatively correlated. Phrased differently, given a relatively inelastic demand curve for health, individuals would desire to offset *part* of the reduction in health capital caused by an increase in the rate of depreciation by increasing their gross investments. In fact, the relationship between the stock of health and the number of healthy days suggests that ε is smaller than one. A general equation for the healthy days production function illustrated by Figure 2 is

$$h_i = 365 - B H_i^{-C}, \tag{2-8}$$

---

[9] That is, $H_{i+1} - H_i \simeq H_i(dH_i/di)(1/H_i) = H_i \tilde{H}_i$. The use of this approximation essentially allows one to ignore the one period lag between a change in gross investment and a change in the stock of health.

[10] Gross investment is nonnegative as long as $I_i = H_i(\tilde{H}_i + \delta_i) \geq 0$, or $\delta_i \geq -\tilde{H}_i$.

where B and C are positive constants. The corresponding MEC schedule is[11]

$$\ln \gamma_i = \ln BC - (C + 1)\ln H_i + \ln W - \ln \pi. \qquad (2\text{-}9)$$

The elasticity of this schedule is given by

$$\varepsilon = -\partial \ln H_i/\partial \ln \gamma_i = 1/(1 + C) < 1,$$

since $C > 0$.

Observe that with the depreciation rate held constant, increases in gross investment would increase the stock of health and the number of healthy days. But the preceding discussion indicates that because the depreciation rate rises with age, it is not unlikely that unhealthy (old) people will make larger gross investments than healthy (young) people. This means that sick time, TL_i, will be positively correlated with M_i and TH_i, the medical care and own time inputs in the gross investment function, over the life cycle.[12] In this sense, at least part of TL_i or TH_i may be termed "recuperation time."

Unlike other models of the demand for medical care, my model does not *assert* that "need" or illness, measured by the level of the rate of depreciation, will definitely be positively correlated with utilization of medical services. Instead, it derives this correlation from the magnitude of the elasticity of the MEC schedule and indicates that the relationship between the stock of health and the number of healthy days will tend to create a positive correlation. If ε is less than one, medical care and "need" will definitely be positively correlated. Moreover, the smaller the value of ε, the greater the explanatory power of "need" relative to that of the other variables in the demand curve for medical care.

It should be realized that the power of this model of life cycle behavior is that it can treat the biological process of aging in terms of conventional economic analysis. Biological factors associated with aging raise the price of health capital and cause individuals to substitute away from future health until death is "chosen." It can be concluded that here, as elsewhere in economics, people will reject a prospect—the prospect

[11] If (2-8) were the production function, the marginal product of health capital would be

$$G_i = BCH_i^{-C-1}, \qquad \text{or} \qquad \ln G_i = \ln BC - (C + 1)\ln H_i.$$

Since $\ln \gamma_i = \ln G_i + \ln W - \ln \pi$, one uses the equation for $\ln G_i$ to obtain (2-9).

[12] Note that the time path of H_i or h_i would be nonmonotonic if the time path of δ_i were characterized by the occurrence of peaks and troughs. In particular, h_i would be relatively low and TH_i and M_i would be relatively high (if $\varepsilon < 1$) when δ_i was relatively high; these periods would be associated with relatively severe illness.

of longer life in this case—because it is too costly to achieve. In particular, only if the elasticity of the MEC schedule were zero would individuals fully compensate for the increase in δ_i and, therefore, maintain a constant stock of health.

Cross-Sectional Variations

The framework used to analyze life cycle variations in depreciation rates can easily be applied to examine the impact of variations in these rates among individuals of the same age. Assume, for example, a uniform percentage shift in δ_i across persons so that

$$\frac{d \ln \delta_{i-1}}{d \ln \delta_i} = 1, \text{ all } i.$$

It is clear that such a shift would have the same kinds of effects as an increase in δ_i with age. That is, persons of a given age who face relatively high depreciation rates would simultaneously reduce their demand for health but would increase their demand for gross investment if $\varepsilon < 1$. Differentiating equations (2-3) and (2-6) with respect to $\ln \delta_i$, one obtains[13]

$$\frac{d \ln H_i}{d \ln \delta_i} = -s_i \varepsilon \tag{2-10}$$

$$\frac{d \ln I_i}{d \ln \delta_i} = \frac{(1 - s_i \varepsilon)(\delta_i - s_i \varepsilon \tilde{\delta}) + s_i^2 \varepsilon \tilde{\delta}}{\delta_i - s_i \varepsilon \tilde{\delta}}. \tag{2-11}$$

According to (2-10) and (2-11), if ε were less than unity, H_i or h_i would be negatively correlated with TH_i and M_i (and TL_i would be positively correlated with these inputs) across individuals of the same age.

Uncertainty

The development of the model to this point has ruled out uncertainty. Consumers fully anticipate intertemporal and cross-sectional variations in depreciation rates and, therefore, know their age of death with certainty. In the real world, however, length of life is surely not known with perfect foresight. In order to explain variations in death time expectations, uncertainty must be introduced into the model. The easiest way to accomplish this is to postulate that a given consumer faces a probability

---

[13] Derivations of (2-10) and (2-11) are contained in Appendix B, Section 2.

distribution of depreciation rates in every period. For simplicity, let there be two depreciation rates, δ_{ia} and δ_{ib}, where $\delta_{ia} > \delta_{ib}$.[14] These depreciation rates correspond to two mutually exclusive outcomes, a and b. Since depreciation rates are not known with certainty, length of life can no longer be determined in a precise fashion. In particular, it would depend on the pattern of depreciation rates that actually occurs and would tend to be longer with patterns in which outcome b occurred more frequently than outcome a. But because depreciation rates rise with age, the stock of health would still tend to fall over the life cycle.

Besides creating dispersion in death time expectations, the existence of uncertainty has a number of additional implications. These follow from the state-preference approach to the problem of choice under uncertainty.[15] Since none of the major conclusions reached in this section and the next one tend to be altered, I will simply state here the main results of the analysis.[16] At any given age, health capital would tend to be lower and sick time and gross investment would tend to be higher in relatively undesirable "states of the world," i.e., outcomes with higher than average depreciation rates. The monetary value of the excess sick time and gross investment measures the "loss" associated with unfavorable states. Since this loss could be reduced by increasing the stock of health, consumers might have an incentive to hold excess stocks in relatively desirable states. In these states, the rate of return to an increase in H_i might be less than the cost of capital. Put differently, part of the demand for health capital would reflect a demand for self-insurance against losses in unfavorable states.

Consumers could also finance the monetary value of their losses by purchasing health insurance in the market. Conclusions reached by Ehrlich and Becker suggest that market health insurance and the stock of health should be substitutes; that is, an increase in market insurance

---

[14] In general, $\delta_{i+1a} > \delta_{ia}$ and $\delta_{i+1b} > \delta_{ib}$ since depreciation rates rise with age.

[15] This approach was developed by Jack Hirshleifer in "Investment Decisions under Uncertainty: Choice-Theoretic Approaches," *Quarterly Journal of Economics*, 79, No. 4 (November 1965). For an application to some general insurance problems, see Isaac Ehrlich and Gary S. Becker, "Market Insurance, Self-Insurance and Self-Protection," *Journal of Political Economy*, 80, No. 4 (July/August 1972).

[16] For derivations of these results, see Michael Grossman, "The Demand for Health: A Theoretical and Empirical Investigation," unpublished Ph.D. dissertation, Columbia University, 1970, Appendix B, pp. 131–135. Note that the assumption of perfect certainty is reintroduced at the end of this subsection. The empirical implementation of the model makes some attempt, however, to deal with uncertainty. See the discussion of this phenomenon in Chapter IV, Section 2, and Chapter V, Section 1.

would increase the optimal loss and reduce the stock of health.[17] Note finally that it is doubtful whether consumers can ever fully insure against all losses via the market. This follows because full insurance would not only finance the monetary value of excess gross investment and working time lost in states with high depreciation rates, but would also finance the monetary value of time lost from nonmarket activities. Hence, the demand for health capital may be substantial even when market insurance is available.

3. MARKET AND NONMARKET EFFICIENCY

Persons who face the same cost of health capital would demand the same amount of health only if the determinants of the rate of return on an investment were held constant. Changes in the value of the marginal product of health capital and the marginal cost of gross investment shift the MEC schedule and, therefore, alter the quantity of health demanded even if the cost of capital does not change. I now identify the variables that determine the level of the MEC schedule and examine the effects of shifts in these variables on the demand for health and medical care.

Before beginning the analysis, two preliminary comments are in order. First, most of the discussion pertains to uniform shifts in variables that influence the rate of return across persons of the same age. That is, if the variable X_i is one determinant, then

$$\frac{d \ln X_i}{d \ln X_{i-1}} = 1, \text{ all } l.$$

Second, the discussion (through equation 2-20) proceeds under the assumption that the real rate of interest, the rate of depreciation, and the elasticity of the MEC schedule are constant. These two comments imply that an increase in X_i will alter the amount of capital demanded but will not alter its rate of change over the life cycle.[18] Note that from equation (2-6)

$$\frac{d \ln I}{dX} = \frac{d \ln H}{dX}, \tag{2-12}$$

---

[17] See Ehrlich and Becker, "Market Insurance."

[18] Strictly speaking, shifts in Y_i would definitely have no effects on $\tilde{H}_i$ if and only if $\tilde{X}_i = 0$. Even though a uniform shift in X_i implies there is no correlation between its level and rate of change, $\tilde{H}_i$ might be altered if $\tilde{X}_i \neq 0$. For a complete discussion, see footnote 30.

since the rate of depreciation and the percentage rate of net investment do not depend on X.[19] Equation (2-12) indicates that percentage changes in health and gross investment for a one unit change in X are identical. Consequently, the effect of an increase in X on either of these two variables can be treated interchangeably.

Wage Effects

Since the value of the marginal product of health capital equals WG, an increase in the wage rate, W, raises the monetary equivalent of the marginal product of a given stock. Put differently, the higher a person's wage rate the greater the value to him of an increase in healthy time. A consumer's wage rate measures his market efficiency or the rate at which he can convert hours of work into money earnings. Hence, it is obviously positively correlated with the benefits of a reduction in the time he loses from the production of money earnings due to illness. Moreover, a high wage rate induces an individual to substitute market goods for his own time in the production of commodities. This substitution continues until in equilibrium the monetary value of the marginal product of consumption time equals the wage rate. So the benefits from a reduction in time lost from nonmarket production are also positively correlated with the wage.

If an upward shift in the wage rate had no effect on the marginal cost of gross investment, a 1 percent increase in it would increase the rate of return, γ, associated with a fixed stock of capital by 1 percent. In fact, this is not the case because own time is an input in the gross investment function. If K is the fraction of the total cost of gross investment accounted for by time, then a 1 percent rise in W would increase marginal cost, π, by K percent. After one nets out the correlation between W and π, the percentage growth in γ would equal $1 - K$, which exceeds zero as long as gross investment is not produced entirely by time.

Since the wage rate and the level of the MEC schedule are positively correlated, the demand for health would be positively related to W. Graphically, an upward shift in W from W_1 to W_2 in Figure 4 shifts the MEC schedule from MEC_1 to MEC_2 and, with no change in the cost of

[19] Since the main part of the analysis in this section deals with variations in X among individuals of the same age, time subscripts are omitted until equation (2-21). Note also that (2-12), like the expression for $\tilde{I}_i$, ignores the one period lag between an increase in gross investment and an increase in the stock of health.

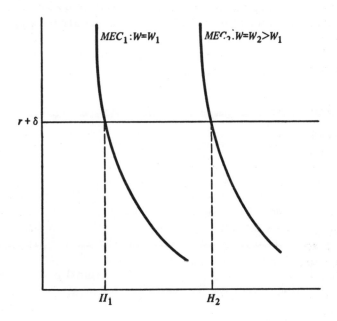

Figure 4

health capital, increases the optimal stock from H_1 to H_2. A formula for the wage elasticity of health capital is[20]

$$e_{H,W} = (1 - K)\varepsilon. \qquad (2\text{-}13)$$

This elasticity is larger the larger the elasticity of the MEC schedule and the larger the share of medical care in total gross investment cost.

Although the wage rate and the demand for health or gross investment are positively related, W has no effect on the amount of gross investment supplied by a given input of medical care. Therefore, the demand for medical care would rise with the wage. If medical care and own time were employed in fixed proportions in the gross investment

[20] Differentiation of the natural logarithm of (2-3) with respect to $\ln W$ yields

$$\frac{d \ln (r + \delta)}{d \ln W} = 0 = 1 + \frac{\partial \ln G}{\partial \ln H} \frac{d \ln H}{d \ln W} - \frac{d \ln \pi}{d \ln W},$$

$$0 = 1 - K - \frac{e_{H,W}}{\varepsilon}.$$

production function, the wage elasticity of M would equal the wage elasticity of H. On the other hand, given a positive elasticity of substitution, M would increase more rapidly than H. This follows because consumers would have an incentive to substitute medical care for their relatively more expensive own time. A formula for the wage elasticity of medical care is

$$e_{M,W} = K\sigma_p + (1 - K)\varepsilon, \qquad\qquad (2\text{-}14)$$

where σ_p is the elasticity of substitution between M and TH in the production of gross investment.[21] The greater the value of σ_p the greater the difference between the wage elasticities of M and H.

Note that an increase in either the price of medical care or own time raises the marginal or average cost of gross investment. But the effects of changes in these two input prices are not symmetrical. In particular, an upward shift in the price of medical care lowers the MEC schedule and causes the demand for health to decline. This difference arises because the price of time influences the value of the marginal product of health capital, while the price of medical care does not.

The Role of Human Capital

Up to now, no systematic allowance has been made for variations in the efficiency of nonmarket production. Yet it is known that firms in the market sector of an economy obtain varying amounts of output from the same vector of direct inputs. These differences have been traced to forces like technology and entrepreneurial capacity, forces that shift production functions or that alter the environment in which the firms operate. Reasoning by analogy, one can say that certain environmental variables influence productivity in the nonmarket sector by altering the marginal products of the direct inputs in household production functions. This study is particularly concerned with environmental variables that can be associated with a particular person—his or her race, sex, stock of human capital, etc.[22] While the analysis that follows could pertain to any

---

[21] For a proof, see Appendix B, Section 2. The corresponding equation for the wage elasticity of TH is

$$e_{TH,W} = (1 - K)(\varepsilon - \sigma_p).$$

This elasticity is positive only if $\varepsilon > \sigma_p$.

[22] Recall from Chapter I that at an operational level the stock of knowledge or human capital does not include health capital.

environmental variable, it is well documented that the more educated are more efficient producers of money earnings. Consequently, it is assumed that shifts in human capital, measured by education, change productivity in the household as well as in the market, and the analysis focuses on this environmental variable.

The specific hypothesis to be tested is that education improves non-market productivity. If this were true, then one would have a convenient way to analyze and quantify what have been termed the nonmonetary benefits to an investment in education. The model can, however, treat adverse as well as beneficial effects and suggests empirical tests to discriminate between the two.[23]

To determine the effects of education on production, marginal cost, and the demand for health and medical care, assume the gross investment production function is homogeneous of degree one in its two direct inputs—medical care and own time. Then the marginal product of E, the index of human capital, would be

$$\frac{\partial I}{\partial E} = M\frac{\partial(g - tg')}{\partial E} + TH\frac{\partial g'}{\partial E},$$

where $g - tg'$ is the marginal product of medical care and g' is the marginal product of time.[24] If a circumflex over a variable denotes a percentage change per unit change in E, the last equation can be rewritten as

$$r_H = \frac{\partial I}{\partial E}\frac{1}{I} = \left[\frac{M(g - tg')}{I}\right]\left[\frac{g\hat{g} - tg'\hat{g}'}{g - tg'}\right] + \left[\frac{THg'}{I}\right][\hat{g}']. \quad (2\text{-}15)$$

Equation (2-15) indicates that the percentage change in gross investment supplied to a consumer by a one unit change in E is a weighted average

---

[23] The model developed here is somewhat similar to the one used by Robert T. Michael in *The Effect of Education on Efficiency in Consumption*, New York, NBER, Occasional Paper 116, 1972. Michael's model examines the effects of education on the demand for consumption commodities and not investment commodities. His analysis, therefore, is more relevant to the consumption model of health presented in Chapter III.

[24] If I is homogeneous of degree one in M and TH, then from Euler's theorem

$$I = M(g - tg') + THg',$$

Differentiation of this equation with respect to E holding M and TH constant yields the marginal product of human capital.

of the percentage changes in the marginal products of M and TH.[25] If E increases productivity, then $r_H > 0$. Provided E raises both marginal products by the same percentage, equation (2-15) would simplify to

$$r_H = \hat{g} = \hat{g}'. \qquad (2\text{-}16)$$

In this case, education would have a "neutral" impact on the marginal products of all factors. The rest of the discussion assumes "factor-neutrality."

Because education raises the marginal product of the direct inputs, it reduces the quantity of these inputs required to produce a given amount of gross investment. Hence, with no change in input prices, an increase in E lowers average or marginal cost. In fact, one easily shows

$$\hat{\pi} = -r_H = -\hat{g} = -\hat{g}', \qquad (2\text{-}17)$$

where $\hat{\pi}$ is the percentage change in average or marginal cost.[26] So if education increases the marginal products of medical care and own time by 3 percent, it would reduce the price of gross investment by 3 percent.

Suppose education does in fact raise productivity so that π and E are negatively correlated. Then with the wage rate and the marginal product of a given stock of health held constant, an increase in education would raise the marginal efficiency of health capital and shift the MEC schedule to the right. In Figure 5, an increase in E from E_1 to E_2 shifts the MEC curve from MEC_1 to MEC_2. If the cost of capital were independent of E, there would be no change in the supply curve, and the more educated would demand a larger optimal stock (compare H_1 and H_2 in the figure). Note that E shifts the MEC schedule not because it is a determinant of consumers' "tastes" for health but because it is a determinant of nonmarket productivity.

[25] Instead of putting education in the gross investment production function, one could let it affect the rate of depreciation or the marginal productivity of health capital. This approach has not been taken because a general treatment of environmental variables like education must permit these variables to influence all household commodities. Since depreciation rates and stock-flow relationships are relevant only if a particular commodity is durable, a symmetrical development of the role of environmental variables requires that they affect household production functions and not depreciation rates or stock-flow relationships. In a more complicated version of the model, the gross investment function, the rate of depreciation, and the marginal productivity of health capital might all depend on education. But the basic implications of the model would not change.

[26] For a proof, see Appendix B, Section 2, where the human capital formulas are developed in more detail.

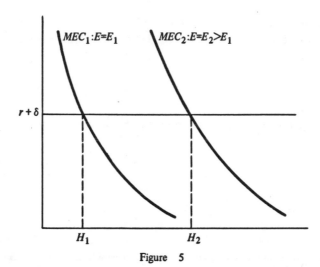

Figure 5

The percentage increase in the amount of health demanded for a one unit increase in E is given by[27]

$$\hat{H} = r_H \varepsilon. \tag{2-18}$$

Since r_H indicates the percentage increase in gross investment supplied by a one unit increase in E, shifts in this variable would not alter the demand for medical care or own time if r_H equaled $\hat{H}$. For example, a person with ten years of formal schooling might demand 3 percent more health than a person with nine years. If the medical care and own time inputs were held constant, the former individual's one extra year of schooling might supply him with 3 percent more health. Given this condition, both persons would demand the same amounts of M and TH. As this example illustrates, any effect of a change in E on the demand for medical care or time reflects a positive or negative differential between $\hat{H}$ and r_H.[28]

$$\hat{M} = \widehat{TH} = r_H(\varepsilon - 1). \tag{2-19}$$

[27] If W and $r + \delta$ are fixed and if G depends only on H, then

$$\frac{d \ln (r + \delta)}{dE} = 0 = \frac{\partial \ln G}{\partial \ln H} \frac{d \ln H}{dE} - \frac{d \ln \pi}{dE}$$

or

$$0 = -\frac{\hat{H}}{\varepsilon} + r_H.$$

[28] The terms $\hat{M}$ and $\widehat{TH}$ are equal because, by the definition of factor neutrality, E has no effect on the ratio of the marginal product of M to the marginal product of TH.

Equation (2-19) suggests that if the elasticity of the MEC schedule were less than unity, the more educated would demand more health but less medical care. Put differently, they would have an incentive to offset *part* of the increase in health caused by an increase in education by reducing their purchases of medical services. Note that if r_H were negative and ε were less than one, $\hat{H}$ would be negative and $\hat{M}$ would be positive Since education improves market productivity, this study tests the hypothesis that r_H is positive. But the model is applicable whether r_H is positive or negative and gives empirical predictions in either case.

Joint Effects

This section has examined the *partial* effect of an increase in the wage rate or an increase in education on the demand for health. But, surely, these two variables are positively correlated, which raises two questions. First, what is the combined effect of an expansion in education, one that takes account of the impact of education on wage rates? Second, can variations in nonmarket efficiency be separated empirically from variations in market efficiency?

A formula for $\hat{H}$ that combines market and nonmarket efficiency changes is

$$\hat{H} = r_H\varepsilon + (1 - K)\varepsilon\hat{W}, \qquad (2\text{-}20)$$

where $\hat{W}$ is the percentage change in the wage rate for a one unit change in E.[29] Equation (2-20) reveals the dual motive of the more educated for demanding more health capital. With nonmarket productivity constant, an increase in E causes the demand price of health capital to rise at a faster rate than the supply price, and with market productivity constant, E is negatively correlated with the supply price. Integration of (2-20) with respect to E yields

$$\ln H = r_H\varepsilon E + (1 - K)\varepsilon \ln W,$$

[29] If W is not held constant as E increases, then

$$\frac{d\ln(r + \delta)}{dE} = 0 = \frac{d\ln W}{dE} + \frac{\partial \ln G}{\partial \ln H}\frac{d\ln H}{dE} - \frac{\partial \ln \pi}{\partial E} - \frac{\partial \ln \pi}{\partial \ln W}\frac{d\ln W}{dE},$$

or

$$0 = W(1 - K) - \frac{\hat{H}}{\varepsilon} + r_H.$$

provided r_H, ε, and K are constant. Hence, by regressing $\ln H$ on E and $\ln W$, *partial* market and nonmarket efficiency parameters can be estimated. Of course, this procedure may break down if the correlation between E and $\ln W$ is extremely high. So it is the size of this correlation that ultimately determines whether pure changes in nonmarket productivity can be isolated at the empirical level.

Along similar lines, the analysis of life cycle variations in the demand for health can be modified to take account of the life cycle pattern of the stock of human capital. Letting $\dot{E}_i = dE_i/di$, one would revise the formula for $\tilde{H}_i$ as follows:[30]

$$\tilde{H}_i = -s_i \varepsilon \tilde{\delta} + r_H \varepsilon \dot{E}_i + (1 - K)\varepsilon \hat{W} \dot{E}_i. \qquad (2\text{-}21)$$

If equation (2-21) were applied to individuals who had completed their formal schooling, E would tend to increase at early ages due to on-the-job training. Eventually it would, however, decline as depreciation on the stock of human capital began to outweigh gross investment. Even if $\tilde{\delta}$ were always positive, the positive values of $\dot{E}_i$ at early stages of the life cycle might make $\tilde{H}_i$ positive during these stages. But ultimately the

---

[30] Replace equation (2-1) with its continuous time analogue:

$$\gamma_i = r - \tilde{\pi}_i + \delta_i.$$

Then if E_i is not fixed as i increases,

$$s_i\tilde{\delta} - \frac{\tilde{\pi}_{ii}\delta_i}{s_i} = \frac{d \ln W_i}{dE_i}\frac{dE_i}{di} + \frac{\partial \ln G_i}{\partial \ln H_i}\frac{d \ln H_i}{di} - \frac{\partial \ln \pi_i}{\partial E_i}\frac{dE_i}{di} - \frac{\partial \ln \pi_i}{\partial \ln W_i}\frac{d \ln W_i}{dE_i}\frac{dE_i}{di}$$

$$s_i\tilde{\delta} - \frac{\tilde{\pi}_{ii}\delta_i}{s_i} = \hat{W}_i\dot{E}_i - \frac{\tilde{H}}{\varepsilon} + r_H\dot{E}_i + (1 - K)\hat{W}_i\dot{E}_i.$$

Note that since the wage rate varies over the life cycle, $\tilde{\pi}_i$ would not, in general, equal zero. Instead, it would be given by

$$\tilde{\pi}_i = (K_i\hat{W}_i - r_H)\dot{E}_i.$$

The equation in the text assumes that $\tilde{\pi}_{ii} = d\tilde{\pi}_i/di \simeq 0$. If r_H and $\hat{W}_i$ were independent of $\dot{E}_i$,

$$\tilde{\pi}_{ii} = (K_i\hat{W} - r_H)\frac{d\dot{E}_i}{di} + (\dot{E}_i\hat{W})^2\frac{dK_i}{d \ln W_i}.$$

Provided the elasticity of substitution on production equaled unity, the second term on the right-hand side of the equation would equal zero. The first term could be ignored if $d\dot{E}_i/di$ were relatively small or if the difference between $K_i\hat{W}$ and r_H were small.

Note also that even if $\hat{W}_i$ and $\dot{E}_i$ were independent of $\ln W_i$, a uniform percentage shift in wage rates across persons of the same age might alter $\tilde{H}_i$. This follows because it would change K_i and hence the real rate of interest unless the elasticity of substitution in production equaled one.

effect of net disinvestment in human capital would strengthen the effect of a rising depreciation rate.

4. GLOSSARY

A tilde over a variable denotes a percentage time derivative; a circumflex over a variable denotes a percentage change per unit change in E; and a dot over a variable denotes an absolute rate of change over the life cycle.

s_i Share of depreciation in the cost of health capital

ε Elasticity of the MEC schedule

K Fraction of the total cost of gross investment accounted for by time

$e_{H,W}$ Elasticity of H with respect to W

$e_{M,W}$ Elasticity of M with respect to W

σ_p Elasticity of substitution between medical care and own time in the production of gross investment

r_H Percentage change in gross investment for a one unit change in E

III

THE PURE CONSUMPTION MODEL

In the previous chapter, I explored the effects of variations in the shadow price of health in the context of the pure investment model. These variations were traced in turn to shifts in the rate of depreciation, market efficiency, and nonmarket efficiency. In this chapter, I utilize the pure consumption model to examine the effects of age, the wage rate, and education.[1] The purpose of the analysis is to indicate the major differences between the investment and consumption models rather than to develop the latter in detail. Consequently, a formal presentation of the consumption model, including derivations of all formulas, has been relegated to Appendix C.

1. LIFE CYCLE PATTERNS

If the cost of capital were large relative to the monetary rate of return on an investment in health and if $\tilde{\pi}_{i-1} = 0$, all i, then equation (1-13) could be approximated by

$$\frac{Uh_i G_i}{\lambda} = \frac{UH_i}{\lambda} = \frac{\pi(r + \delta_i)}{(1 + r)^i}. \qquad (3\text{-}1)$$

Equation (3-1) indicates that the monetary equivalent of the marginal utility of health capital in period i must equal the discounted user cost of H_i.[2] Division of the equilibrium condition for H_{i+1} by the equilibrium

---

[1] The model of life cycle behavior presented in this chapter is similar to Gilbert R. Ghez's analysis of life cycle demand for durable consumer goods. See "A Theory of Life Cycle Consumption," unpublished Ph.D. dissertation, Columbia University, 1970, Chapter I.

[2] Solving equation (3-1) for the monetary equivalent of the marginal utility of healthy time, one has

$$\frac{Uh_i}{\lambda} = \frac{\pi(r + \delta_i)/G_i}{(I + r)^i},$$

where $\pi(r + \delta_i)/G_i$ is the undiscounted price of a healthy day. Given diminishing marginal productivity of health capital, this price would be positively correlated with H or h even if π were constant. Therefore, the consumption demand curve would be influenced by scale effects. To emphasize the main issues at stake in the consumption model, I ignore these scale effects essentially by assuming that ϕ_i and hence G_i are constant. The analysis would not be greatly altered if they were introduced.

condition for H_i generates the basic equation for the analysis of life cycle demand:

$$\frac{UH_{i+1}}{UH_i} = (1 + r)^{-1}\left(\frac{r + \delta_{i+1}}{r + \delta_i}\right). \tag{3-2}$$

Condition (3-2) simply states that the marginal rate of substitution between H_i and H_{i+1} must equal the ratio of the discounted user cost of H_{i+1} to the discounted user cost of H_i.

To characterize the life cycle path of health capital in a precise manner, certain restrictions must be placed on the utility function. In particular, it must be assumed that this function is weakly separable in H_i and H_{i+1}. That is, the marginal rate of substitution between H_i and H_{i+1} depends only on these two stocks and is independent of the other H's and all other commodities. It is also assumed for the present that there is no "health time preference." This means that $UH_{i+1}/UH_i = m = 1$ when $H_{i+1} = H_i$. Of course, since indifference curves are convex to the origin, a reduction in H_{i+1} relative to H_i along a given indifference curve would increase UH_{i+1} relative to UH_i.

Suppose the rate of interest were zero and the rate of depreciation were independent of age. Then the discounted user cost ratio and, therefore, the marginal rate of substitution between H_i and H_{i+1} would equal unity. Given no time preference, this implies $H_i = H_{i+1}$. If the rate of interest were positive, the discounted user cost ratio and, hence, UH_{i+1}/UH_i would be less than unity. Convexity of indifference curves implies $H_{i+1} > H_i$ in this situation. Therefore, under the stated conditions of no time preference and constant depreciation rates, H_i would rise over time if $r > 0$ and would be stationary if $r = 0$. Either of these two life cycle patterns suggests that individuals would choose to live forever.

As in the investment model, a positive correlation between the rate of depreciation and age generates a stock of health pattern that is consistent with a finite life. To see this, first let the rate of interest equal zero. Then the discounted user cost ratio would equal δ_{i+1}/δ_i, which is clearly greater than one. It follows that UH_{i+1}/UH_i must exceed one, and this implies $H_{i+1} < H_i$. Thus, the stock of health would fall throughout the life cycle because the price of the next period's health in terms of its present period price is always greater than one.

Now let the rate of interest be positive. In this case, H_{i+1} might exceed H_i even if $\delta_{i+1} > \delta_i$. But if δ_i grew at a constant rate, the discounted user cost ratio would rise over time.[3] Since this price ratio increases over time, so must the marginal rate of substitution between H_{i+1} and H_i. Convexity of indifference curves dictates that H_{i+1}/H_i must fall with age. Health capital might increase for a while but would peak when the depreciation effect began to outweigh the interest rate effect. After the peak is reached, H_i would decline until death is "chosen."

A formula for the percentage rate of change in health capital over the life cycle is given by[4]

$$\tilde{H}_i = \sigma[\ln m + \ln(1 + r) - s_i\tilde{\delta}]. \tag{3-3}$$

In this formula, σ is the elasticity of substitution in consumption between H_i and H_{i+1}:

$$\sigma = \frac{\partial(\ln H_i/H_{i+1})}{\partial(\ln UH_{i+1}/UH_i)}.$$

Equation (3-3) includes a time preference effect as well as interest and depreciation effects. If there were time preference for the present, the marginal utility of H_i would exceed the marginal utility of H_{i+1} when $H_i = H_{i+1}$. Hence $\ln m < 0$, and H_i would fall faster and death would occur sooner given preference for the present. On the other hand, preference for the future makes $\ln m > 0$ and prolongs the time interval during which H increases. Equation (3-3) also indicates that H_i reaches its maximum quantity when $\ln m + \ln(1 + r) = s_i\tilde{\delta}$.[5]

Although the demand for health capital declines after some point in the life cycle, gross investment would tend to be positively correlated with age if the elasticity of substitution between present and future health were less than unity.[6] Put differently, if present and future health were relatively poor substitutes, individuals would have an incentive to

---

[3] If $\tilde{\delta}$ were constant, then the derivative of the natural logarithm of the discounted user cost ratio would be

$$\tilde{\delta}\left[\frac{r(\delta_{i+1} - \delta_i)}{(r + \delta_i)(r + \delta_{i+1})}\right] > 0,$$

since $\delta_{i+1} > \delta_i$.

[4] For a derivation of equation (3-3), see Appendix C, Section 1.

[5] When $\ln m + \ln(1 + r) = s_i\tilde{\delta}$, $\tilde{H}_i = 0$. This stationary point gives a maximum since $\tilde{H}_{ii} < 0$:

$$\tilde{H}_{ii} = -s_i(1 - s_i)\sigma\tilde{\delta}^2.$$

The formula for $\tilde{H}_{ii}$ assumes σ and $\tilde{\delta}$ are constant.

[6] For a proof, see Appendix C, Section 1.

offset part of the reduction in health caused by an increase in the rate of depreciation by increasing their gross investments. In fact, there is reason to believe that the elasticity of substitution is relatively small, at least in the vicinity of the death stock. To see why this is the case, redefine σ as

$$\sigma = \frac{\partial(\ln H'_i/H'_{i+1})}{\partial(\ln UH'_{i+1}/UH'_i)},$$

where $H'_i = H_i - H_{min}$.[7] I have shown that H'_i/H'_{i+1} rises with age, which increases UH'_{i+1}/UH'_i. Since $UH'_{i+1}/UH'_i \to \infty$ as $H'_{i+1} \to 0$ and since this condition must be satisfied at death, small increases in H'_i/H'_{i+1} must have large effects on the ratio of marginal utilities around the death age.[8]

In both the consumption and investment models, biological factors associated with aging cause individuals to substitute away from future health until death is chosen. There are two major differences between the two models. First, even if the depreciation rate rises continuously with age, the existence of time preference for the future or a positive rate of interest might cause health capital to increase for a while in the consumption model. Second, the elasticity of substitution between present and future health, rather than the elasticity of the MEC schedule, determines (1) the responsiveness of health to a change in the rate of depreciation and (2) the life cycle behavior of gross investment.

2. MARKET AND NONMARKET EFFICIENCY

To study the effects of variations in the shadow price of health among individuals of the same age, a cross-sectional consumption demand curve must be specified. The simplest specification is

$$H = H(R^*, Q^*), \tag{3-4}$$

where $R^* = R/Q$, real full wealth; $Q^* = \pi(r + \delta)/Q$, the relative user cost or shadow price of health; $\ln Q = w \ln \pi(r + \delta) + (1 - w) \ln q$, the natural logarithm of a weighted geometric price level of health and the

[7] This definition implies the death time utility function is

$$U = U(\phi_i H'_i, Z_i).$$

If both consumption and investment aspects of the demand for health were considered, H'_i and Z_i would equal zero at death. Hence, total utility would be driven to zero provided $U(0, 0) = 0$.

[8] If the elasticity of substitution were constant, it would have to be small at all stages of the life cycle and not just in the vicinity of the death stock.

aggregate commodity Z, where the weights w and $(1 - w)$ are shares of these commodities in full wealth, and where q is the price of Z. A reduction in the relative shadow price of health would lead consumers to substitute H for the aggregate commodity Z. Moreover, if health were not an inferior commodity, an increase in real full wealth would increase demand. The magnitudes of responses in H to changes in relative price and real wealth are summarized by e_H, the own price elasticity of demand, and η_H, the wealth elasticity.

Wage Effects

Differentiation of equation (3-4) with respect to the wage rate yields[9]

$$e_{H,W} = -e_H(K - \bar{K}).\qquad(3-5)$$

In this equation, K is the fraction of the total cost of gross investment accounted for by time and $\bar{K}$ is the average time intensity of nonmarket production. The derivation of (3-5) holds real wealth constant so that the equation shows the pure substitution effect of a change in the wage rate. Since e_H is positive by definition, $e_{H,W} \lesseqgtr 0$ as $K \gtreqless \bar{K}$.

The sign of the wage elasticity is ambiguous because an increase in the wage raises the marginal cost of gross investment in health and the marginal cost of Z. Hence, both π and the price level are positively correlated with W. If time costs were relatively more important in the production of health than in the production of a typical nonmarket commodity, the relative price of health would rise with the wage rate, which would reduce the quantity demanded. The ambiguity of the wage effect here is in sharp contrast to the situation in the investment model. In that model, the wage rate would be positively correlated with health as long as K were less than one.

The Role of Human Capital

To study the effects of variations in nonmarket productivity associated with education, note that since E influences productivity in all nonmarket activities, it alters the marginal costs of all home-produced commodities. Given factor-neutrality, the percentage reduction in the

---

[9] For a proof, see Appendix C, Section 2. The corresponding equation for the wage elasticity of medical care is

$$e_{M,W} = K\sigma_p - (K - \bar{K})e_H.$$

marginal cost of the aggregate commodity Z would be $-r_Z$, where r_Z is the percentage increase in either the marginal product of Z's goods input or time input as E increases. Therefore, human capital's effect on the weighted geometric price level is given by

$$\hat{Q} = -r_E = -[wr_H + (1 - w)r_Z].$$

With money full wealth fixed, the term r_E can be viewed as the percentage change in real full wealth due to the change in nonmarket productivity associated with education. It indicates the nonmonetary return to an investment in education.[10]

If education improved productivity, then the last equation suggests that an increase in this variable would reduce the absolute shadow prices of all home-produced commodities, increase real wealth, and also alter relative prices provided the improvements in productivity were not the same for all commodities. Therefore, a shift in E would set in motion wealth and substitution effects that would alter the demand for health. Differentiating the demand function (3-4) with respect to E, holding money full wealth and the wage rate constant, one obtains[11]

$$\hat{H} = r_E\eta_H + e_H(r_H - r_E). \tag{3-6}$$

The first term on the right-hand side of equation (3-6) reflects the wealth effect, and the second term reflects the substitution effect. If E's productivity effect on the gross investment function were the same as its average productivity effect, then $r_H = r_E$, and $\hat{H}$ would reflect the wealth effect alone. In this situation, a shift in education would be "commodity-neutral." If $r_H > r_E$, E would be "biased" toward health, its relative price would fall, and the wealth and substitution effects would both operate in the same direction. Consequently, an increase in E would definitely increase the demand for health. If $r_H < r_E$, E would be biased away from health, its relative price would rise, and the wealth and substitution effects would operate in opposite directions.

The human capital parameter in the demand curve for medical care is given by

$$\hat{M} = r_E(\eta_H - 1) + (r_H - r_E)(e_H - 1). \tag{3-7}$$

[10] For an exhaustive discussion of the above method of specifying the nonmonetary benefits of education, see Robert T. Michael, *The Effect of Education on Efficiency in Consumption*, New York, NBER, Occasional Paper 116, 1972, Chap. 1.

[11] For derivations of the human capital parameters given by equations (3-6) and (3-7), see Appendix C, Section 2.

If shifts in E were "commodity-neutral," then medical care and education would be negatively correlated unless $\eta_H \geq 1$. If, on the other hand, there were a bias in favor of health, these two variables would still tend to be negatively correlated unless the wealth and price elasticities both exceeded one.

The preceding discussion reveals that the analysis of variations in nonmarket productivity in the consumption model differs in two important respects from the corresponding analysis in the investment model. In the first place, wealth effects are not relevant in the pure investment model. This follows because an increase in wealth with no change in the interest rate and the rate of depreciation would not alter the equality between the cost of capital and the rate of return on an investment in health. Note that health would have a positive wealth elasticity in the investment model if wealthier people faced lower rates of interest.[12] But the analysis of shifts in education assumes money wealth is fixed. Thus, one could not rationalize the positive relationship between education and health in terms of an association between wealth and the interest rate.

In the second place, if the investment framework were utilized, then whether or not a shift in human capital is commodity-neutral would be irrelevant in assessing its effect on the demand for health. As long as the rate of interest were independent of education, H and E would be positively correlated. Put differently, if individuals could always receive, say, a 5 percent rate of return on savings deposited in a savings bank, then a shift in education would create a gap between the cost of capital and the marginal efficiency of a given stock.

3. GLOSSARY

UH_i Marginal utility of H_i
m Index of time preference
σ Elasticity of substitution between H_{i+1} and H_i
R^* Real full wealth
Q^* Relative user cost or shadow price of health
Q Weighted geometric price level

[12] If the rate of interest depends on full wealth and if health does not enter the utility function, then

$$\eta_H = -(1 - s)\varepsilon\eta_r,$$

where $1 - s$ is the share of interest in the cost of health capital and η_r is the wealth elasticity of the interest rate.

e_H Own price elasticity of demand for health

η_H Wealth elasticity of demand for health

$\overline{K}$ Average time intensity of nonmarket production

r_Z Percentage change in either the marginal product of goods or time in the Z production function for a one unit change in E

r_E Percentage change in real full wealth for a one unit change in E

IV

AN EMPIRICAL FORMULATION OF THE MODEL

In the previous chapters, I have developed a framework that can be employed to predict the effects of certain variables on the demand for health and medical care. To test the implications of this framework, it is necessary to estimate demand curves for health and medical care and perhaps a gross investment production function as well. In the first section of this chapter, I explore the estimation of this set of equations in detail. In particular, I outline the structure and reduced form of the pure investment model. Although the formulation is oriented toward the investment framework, I offer two tests to distinguish the investment model from the consumption model. In the second section, I describe the measures of health used in the empirical analysis, discuss the data source from which these measures are obtained, and comment on the independent variables that enter the multiple regression estimates of the system.

The estimation of the investment model rather than the consumption model is stressed because the former model generates powerful predictions from simple analysis and innocuous assumptions. For example, if one uses the investment framework, then he does not have to know whether the production of health is relatively time-intensive to predict the effect of an increase in the wage rate on the demand for health. Again, he does not have to know whether shifts in education are commodity-neutral to assess the sign of the correlation between health and schooling. Moreover, the responsiveness of the quantity of health demanded to changes in its shadow price and the behavior of gross investment depend essentially on a single parameter—the elasticity of the MEC schedule. In the consumption model, on the other hand, three parameters are relevant—the own price elasticity of health, the elasticity of substitution between present and future health, and the wealth elasticity.

1. STRUCTURE AND REDUCED FORM

To derive estimating equations for the pure investment model, begin with the production function of healthy days utilized in Chapter II:

$$h_i = 365 - BH_i^{-C}. \qquad (4\text{-}1)$$

Although the subscript i refers to age, it should be clear that H will vary across individuals as well as over the life cycle of a given individual. It has already been shown[1] that this production function generates the constant elasticity MEC schedule[2]

$$\ln \gamma_i = \ln BC - (C + 1) \ln H_i + \ln W_i - \ln \pi_i,$$

where $\varepsilon = 1/(1 + C)$. Solving the last equation for $\ln H_i$ and substituting $r - \tilde{\pi}_i + \delta_i$ for γ_i, one obtains the stock of health demand function

$$\ln H_i = B' + \varepsilon \ln W_i - \varepsilon \ln \pi_i - \varepsilon \ln (r - \tilde{\pi}_i + \delta_i), \qquad (4\text{-}2)$$

where $B' = \ln BC/(1 + C)$. Suppose $\tilde{\pi}_i$ is positive and constant and the real-own rate of interest is equal to zero. Then equation (4-1) would reduce to

$$\ln H_i = B' + \varepsilon \ln W_i - \varepsilon \ln \pi_i - \varepsilon \ln \delta_i. \qquad (4\text{-}3)$$

Although age and education do not appear explicitly on the right-hand side of (4-3), they are implicit in this equation because the rate of depreciation and the marginal cost of gross investment are not directly observable and expressions for them must be developed. It has been hypothesized that depreciation rates rise with age, at least after some stage in the life cycle, and vary among individuals of the same age as well. Let these factors be summarized by a depreciation rate equation of the form

$$\ln \delta_i = \ln \delta_0 + \tilde{\delta} i. \qquad (4\text{-}4)$$

An equation for marginal cost can be developed from the household production function for gross investment. For analytical convenience, assume the production function is a member of the Cobb–Douglas class:

$$\ln I_i = r_H E + \alpha_1 \ln M_i + (1 - \alpha_1) \ln TH_i. \qquad (4\text{-}5)$$

Here $\alpha_1 = 1 - K$ is the share of medical care in the total cost of gross investment or the elasticity of gross investment with respect to medical care. With this production function, the elasticity of substitution between medical services and own time equals one. Consequently, K is independent of the prices of these inputs.

---

[1] See Chapter II, footnote 11.

[2] Continuous time equilibrium conditions are utilized in this chapter. Hence, $\gamma_i = W_i G_i/\pi_i$, and the real-own rate of interest is $r - \tilde{\pi}_i$.

Appendix D, Section 1, demonstrates that equations (4-3) and (4-4) generate the following reduced form demand curves for health and medical care:[3]

$$\ln H_i = (1 - K)\varepsilon \ln W_i - K\varepsilon \ln P + r_H \varepsilon E - \tilde{\delta}\varepsilon i - \varepsilon \ln \delta_0, \quad (4\text{-}6)$$

$$\ln M_i = [(1 - K)\varepsilon + K] \ln W_i - [(1 - K)\varepsilon + K] \ln P + r_E(\varepsilon - 1)E$$
$$+ \tilde{\delta}(1 - \varepsilon)i + (1 - \varepsilon) \ln \delta_0 + \ln(1 + H_i/\delta_i). \quad (4\text{-}7)$$

A demand curve for the time spent producing health could also be developed, but data pertaining to this input are, in general, not available. Equations (4-2) and (4-5) may be termed the basic structural relations of the investment model, while equations (4-6) and (4-7) are the ones that will be actually estimated to test the implications of the model. At this point, a number of comments concerning these latter two equations are in order.

If the absolute value of the percentage rate of net disinvestment were small relative to the rate of depreciation, the last term in (4-7) could be ignored.[4] Then (4-6) and (4-7) would express the two main endogenous variables in the system as functions of four variables that are treated as exogenous within the context of this model—the wage rate, the price of medical care, the stock of human capital, and age—and one variable that is unobserved, the rate of depreciation in the initial period. If P, the price of medical care, did not vary across the relevant units of observation, the estimating equations would become

$$\ln H_i = B_W \ln W + B_E E + B_i i + U_1 \quad (4\text{-}6')$$

$$\ln M_i = B_{WM} \ln W + B_{EM} E + B_{iM} i + U_2, \quad (4\text{-}7')$$

where $B_W = \varepsilon(1 - K)$, etc., $U_1 = -\varepsilon \ln \delta_0$, and $U_2 = (1 - \varepsilon) \ln \delta_0$. The investment model predicts $B_W > 0$, $B_E > 0$, $B_i < 0$, and $B_{WM} > 0$. In addition, if $\varepsilon < 1$, $B_{EM} < 0$, and $B_{iM} > 0$.

The variables U_1 and U_2 represent disturbance terms in the reduced form equations. These terms are present because depreciation rates vary among individuals of the same age, and such variations cannot be measured empirically. Provided $\ln \delta_0$ were not correlated with the independent variables in (4-6') and (4-7'), U_1 and U_2 would not be

[3] Equations (4-5), (4-6), and (4-7) do not contain intercepts because all variables are expressed as deviations from their respective means.

[4] Chapter II indicated that if the stock of health falls over the life cycle, then the rate of depreciation must exceed the absolute value of the rate of net disinvestment. From equation (4-6), $\tilde{H}_i = -\tilde{\delta}\varepsilon < 0$. If $\tilde{H}_i$ is small relative to δ_i, $\tilde{H}_i/\delta_i$ approaches zero.

correlated with these variables. Therefore, the equations could be estimated by ordinary least squares.

The assumption that the real-own rate of interest equals zero can be justified along the following lines. A common empirical observation is that wage rates rise with age, at least during most stages of the life cycle. If W_i were growing at a constant rate $\tilde{W}$, then $\tilde{\pi}_i = K\tilde{W}$, all i. So the assumption implies $r = K\tilde{W}$. By eliminating the real rate of interest and postulating that $\tilde{H}_i$ is small relative to δ_i, $\ln H_i$ and $\ln M_i$ are made linear functions of age. If $r - \tilde{\pi}_i$ exceeded zero but $\tilde{H}_i/\delta_i$ were small, then

$$\tilde{H}_i = -\tilde{\delta}s_i\varepsilon$$
$$\tilde{M}_i = \tilde{\delta}(1 - s_i\varepsilon)$$
$$\tilde{H}_{ii} = \tilde{M}_{ii} = -\tilde{\delta}^2 s_i(1 - s_i)\varepsilon.$$

Since the curves relating $\ln H_i$ and $\ln M_i$ to age would be concave to the origin in this situation, the square of age might be included as an additional explanatory variable. This variable should have negative coefficients in the demand curves for health and medical care.

One could change the form of the gross investment production function without altering any of the parameters in (4-6) and (4-7) except the wage elasticity of medical care. For example, suppose medical care and own time were employed in fixed proportions. Then the elasticity of substitution between these two inputs would equal zero, and the wage elasticities of health and medical care would be equal.

There are two empirical procedures for assessing whether the investment model gives a more adequate representation of people's behavior than the consumption model. In the first place, the wage rate would have a positive effect on the demand for health in the investment model as long as K were less than one. On the other hand, it would have a positive effect in the consumption model only if health were relatively goods-intensive ($K < \bar{K}$), a somewhat more restrictive requirement. So if the computed wage elasticity turns out to be positive, then the larger its value the more likely it is that the investment model is preferable to the consumption model. Of course, provided the production of health were relatively time-intensive, the wage elasticity would be negative in the consumption model. In this case, a positive and statistically significant estimate of B_W would lead to a rejection of the consumption model.

In the second place, suppose the rate of interest does not depend on wealth. Then health would have a zero wealth elasticity in the investment model. It would, however, have a positive wealth elasticity in the consumption model if it is a superior commodity. This suggests that $\ln R$, the logarithm of full wealth, should be added to the set of independent variables in the demand curves for health and medical care so that these equations would become

$$\ln H_i = B_R \ln R + B_W \ln W + B_E E + B_i i + U_1 \qquad (4\text{-}6'')$$

$$\ln M_i = B_{RM} \ln R + B_{WM} \ln W + B_{EM} E + B_{iM} i + U_2. \quad (4\text{-}7'')$$

Computed wealth elasticities of H and M that do not differ significantly from zero would tend to support the investment model. Although the investment framework could rationalize positive wealth elasticities in terms of a negative correlation between R and r,[5] this correlation is not likely to be very large. Regardless of the size of the correlation between R and r, the wealth effect would be small if the share of depreciation in the cost of health capital were relatively large.[6]

In addition to fitting equations (4-6'') and (4-7'') to the data, the gross investment function given by equation (4-5) might also be estimated. By estimating the production function, the hypothesis that the more educated are more efficient producers of health could be tested directly. Note that the production function contains two variables for which no data exist—gross investment and the own time input. But since $\ln I_i = \ln H_i + \ln (\tilde{H}_i + \delta_i)$ and since $\tilde{H}_i/\delta_i$ has been assumed to be small, one could fit[7]

$$\ln H_i = \alpha \ln M_i + r_H E - \tilde{\delta}_i i - \ln \delta_0. \qquad (4\text{-}8)$$

The trouble with the above procedure is that it requires a good estimate of the gross investment production function. Unfortunately, equation (4-8) cannot be fitted by ordinary least squares because $\ln M_i$ and $\ln \delta_0$, the disturbance term, are bound to be correlated. It is clear from the demand curve for medical care that

$$\text{Cov} (\ln M_i, \ln \delta_0) = (1 - \varepsilon)\sigma^2 \ln \delta_0,$$

[5] In addition, the real rate of interest would have to be positive.

[6] Health would also have a positive wealth elasticity in the investment model for people who are not in the labor force. For such individuals, an increase in wealth would raise the ratio of market goods to consumption time, the marginal productivity of consumption time, and its shadow price. Hence, the monetary rate of return on an investment in health would increase. Since the empirical work in the next section is limited to members of the labor force, a pure increase in wealth would not change the shadow price of their time.

[7] If factor prices do not vary as more and more health is produced, a 1 percent increase in medical care would be accompanied by an equal percentage increase in own time. Therefore, the regression coefficient α in equation (4-7) would reflect the elasticity of gross investment or health capital with respect to both inputs. Given constant returns to scale, the true value of α should be unity.

where Cov means covariance and $\sigma^2 \ln \delta_0$ is the variance of $\ln \delta_0$. So, given $\varepsilon < 1, \ln M_i$ and $\ln \delta_0$ would be positively correlated. Since an increase in the rate of depreciation decreases the quantity of health capital demanded, the coefficient of medical care would be biased *downward*. If wealth were included in the set of exogenous variables, the production function would be "overidentified" and could be fitted by two-stage least squares.[8] Using this technique, one would first estimate the demand curve for medical care. He would then compute the predicted values of $\ln M$, which by definition are not correlated with $\ln \delta_0$. Finally, he would use these predicted values to estimate the production function.

While the two-stage least squares technique is employed in the next chapter, there are a number of difficulties with it and major reliance is placed on the calculations of the reduced form. These difficulties are discussed when the production function estimates are presented. A production function taken by itself tells nothing about producer or consumer behavior, although it does have implications for behavior, which operate on the demand curves for health and medical care. Thus, they serve to rationalize the forces at work in the reduced form and give the variables that enter the equations economic significance. Because the reduced form parameters can be used to explain consumer choices and because they can be obtained by conventional statistical techniques, their interpretation should be pushed as far as possible. Only then should one resort to a direct estimate of the production function.

2. MEASUREMENT OF HEALTH AND VARIABLES CONSIDERED

The equations formulated in Section 1 have been fitted to data contained in the 1963 health interview survey conducted by the National Opinion Research Center and the Center for Health Administration Studies of the University of Chicago. The NORC sample is an area probability sample of the civilian noninstitutionalized population in which each family had the same probability of inclusion. Data were obtained from 2,367 families containing 7,803 persons.[9]

[8] The production function is overidentified because the number of variables excluded from it (R and W) exceeds the number of endogenous variables in the system (H and M) less one by a factor of one. If wealth were not an endogenous variable, the number of excluded variables would equal the number of endogenous variables less one. In this situation, the production function would be "exactly identified" and could still be estimated by two-stage least squares.

[9] For a complete description of the sample, see Ronald Andersen and Odin W. Anderson, *A Decade of Health Services: Social Survey Trends in Use and Expenditure*, Chicago, 1967.

The stock of health, like the stock of knowledge, is a theoretical concept, one that is difficult to quantify empirically. On the other hand, the healthy time output produced by health capital can be measured in a straightforward fashion. If TL_i is time (in days) lost from market and non-market activities due to illness and injury, then $h_i = 365 - TL_i$. Therefore, consider the results that would be obtained if healthy time or its complement served as the dependent variable in the demand curve. The production function of healthy days given by equation (4-1) implies

$$- \ln TL_i = - \ln B + C \ln H_i. \tag{4-9}$$

Substitution of equation (4-6) for $\ln H_i$ yields[10]

$$-\ln TL_i = CB_R \ln R + C(1 - K)\varepsilon \ln W_i + Cr_H \varepsilon E - C\tilde{\delta}\varepsilon i - C\varepsilon \ln \delta_0. \tag{4-10}$$

While equation (4-6) gives a demand curve for the stock of health, equation (4-10) gives a demand curve for the flow of services yielded by health capital. The flow coefficients can be estimated by regressing the negative of the natural logarithm of sick time on the relevant set of exogenous variables. The coefficients obtained would exceed, equal, or fall short of the corresponding coefficients in the stock demand curve as C exceeds, equals, or falls short of 1. The formulation of the flow demand curve suggests that $-\ln TL_i$, and not $\ln h_i$, should be the dependent variable. Consequently, the increase in healthy time for a one unit increase in education *falls* as education increases.[11] Thus, although education has an increasing marginal product in the gross investment production function, the model still implies diminishing returns to this variable in terms of its impact on healthy time.

Two variants of sick time are available in the NORC sample. These are the number of restricted-activity days reported by persons in 1963 and the number of work-loss days. A restricted-activity day (RAD) is a day on which a person is kept away from his usual activities because of

---

[10] The derivation of (4-10) assumes that wealth is one of the independent variables in (4-6). In addition, all variables are expressed as deviations from their respective means.

[11] Let $\hat{B} = Cr_H\varepsilon$. Then from equation (4-10),

$$\frac{\partial h}{\partial E} = \hat{B} \exp(-\hat{B}E),$$

and

$$\frac{\partial^2 h}{\partial E^2} = -\hat{B}^2 \exp(-\hat{B}E) < 0.$$

illness or injury. A work-loss day (WLD) is a day on which a person would have gone to work but instead lost the entire day because of illness or injury. Work-loss days are, of course, relevant only for members of the labor force. For such individuals, every WLD is an RAD, but the converse is not true. This follows because an RAD might occur on a Saturday, Sunday, holiday, or vacation day or because an individual might go to work even though he does not feel well but might cut down on his nonmarket activities.

Although RAD is a more encompassing measure of sick time than WLD, both variables have been employed because it seems likely that the latter is a more objective concept than the former. In other words, respondents can probably recall and identify WLD with more precision than they can recall and identify RAD. To compare the results obtained with the two measures, only members of the labor force are included in the regressions computed with the NORC sample. The labor force consists of all people who reported their current status on the date the sample was taken (early 1964) as working full time, working part time, or unemployed. People who fell into one of these three categories but who failed to report the number of weeks they worked in 1963 or who said they worked no weeks in that year were excluded from the regressions.

At this point, it will be useful to discuss four methodological issues that arise when the complement of sick days, and especially when the complement of WLD, is used as a measure of the services yielded by the stock of health. First, part of the variation in WLD might simply reflect variations in weeks worked among individuals. To cite a rather extreme example, someone who worked only one week in 1963 might have reported many fewer work-loss days than someone who worked fifty weeks. If weeks worked were correlated with some of the independent variables in (4-10), the estimates of the parameters of this equation would be biased. To take account of this problem, WLD is adjusted for variations in weeks worked (WW).[12] Adjusted WLD is given by[13]

$$WLD1 = (52/WW)(WLD).$$

Second, sick time should not be confused with the time input in the gross investment function. In Chapter II, I pointed out that in the absence

[12] Weeks worked are defined as weeks actually worked plus paid vacation time plus work-loss weeks.

[13] The correlation coefficient between unadjusted and adjusted work-loss is .97. Regression coefficients obtained with unadjusted work-loss as the dependent variable (not shown) are very similar to the coefficients presented in the next chapter.

of variations in depreciation rates, these two variables would be *negatively* correlated. I also demonstrated that if depreciation rates did vary, the correlation might well be *positive*. But provided δ_0 were independent of the exogenous variables in (4-10), the coefficients of this equation could be interpreted in the manner that has been suggested.[14]

A third methodological issue arises if consumers face a probability distribution of depreciation rates in each period of their lives. As stated in Chapter II, individuals who insure against this uncertainty in part by acquiring market insurance would have smaller stocks of health and more sick days than those who rely solely on self-insurance. The latter group protect themselves against potential losses by holding excess stocks in relatively desirable states of the world—excess in the sense that the marginal efficiency of health capital might be extremely small and even zero in some cases. To standardize for the effects of uncertainty, a variable that indicates the presence or absence of disability insurance (insurance that finances earnings lost due to illness or injury) is included in some of the regressions run. This insurance variable might be related to observed sick time not only because of its effect on potential losses but also because of its effect on the probability that a given loss will occur. The theory of "moral hazard" suggests that if the insurance premium paid by an individual is fixed, then he may have an incentive to increase his probability of loss.[15]

Finally, some investigators have argued that the number of work-loss days reported by a person is determined almost entirely by the presence or absence of disability insurance and informal sick leave arrangements. These investigators claim that to a large extent, measured work-loss is simply one component of "leisure time." Hence, this variable is an unreliable indicator of the health status of individuals.[16]

[14] For the contrary view, see Morris Silver, "An Economic Analysis of Variations in Medical Expenses and Work-Loss Rates," in Herbert E. Klarman (ed.), *Empirical Studies in Health Economics*, Baltimore, 1970, and reprinted as Chapter 6 in Victor R. Fuchs (ed.), *Essays in the Economics of Health and Medical Care*, New York, NBER, 1972. Part of Silver's analysis is based on the assumption that sick time and the time input are identical. Suppose δ_0 were correlated with some of the independent variables that Silver and I use in our regressions. Then his view that the two types of time are equivalent would be partially correct, my view that they are different would also be partially correct, and the truth would lie somewhere between these two extremes. The empirical results in the next chapter seem to indicate, however, that my assumption concerning sick time is very plausible.

[15] See Isaac Ehrlich and Gary S. Becker, "Market Insurance, Self-Insurance and Self-Protection," *Journal of Political Economy*, 80, No. 4 (July/August 1972).

[16] For a summary of this argument, see Philip E. Enterline, "Sick Absences in Certain Western Countries," *Industrial Medicine and Surgery*, 33, No. 10 (October 1964).

The NORC data tends to contradict this view since the observed correlation between medical care and sick time is positive and very significant. The correlation between M and $WLD1$ is .356 and the correlation between M and RAD is .409. These correlations reflect the positive relationship between medical care and the depreciation rate. Apparently, this relationship is so strong that it swamps the positive effect of an increase in medical care on health (or the negative effect on sick time) that would be observed if the depreciation rate were held constant. These correlations substantiate the common-sense point of view that illness and utilization of medical services are positively associated. They also indicate that the number of work-loss days reported by the members of the sample measures their illness levels rather than a fraction of their leisure time.

The dependent variable in the demand curve for medical care is personal medical outlays. Medical expenditures include outlays on doctors, dentists, hospital care, prescribed and nonprescribed drugs, nonmedical practitioners, and other medical care—chiefly appliances like eyeglasses. Expenditures exclude health insurance premiums but contain benefits paid for by insurance.

Dollar outlays are a more desirable measure of medical care than quantity indexes for two reasons. First, the former allows one to combine the various components of medical care into an aggregate index of the utilization of this care in a simple way. Second, part of the variation in price across individuals reflects variations in the quality of services purchased instead of true differences in the price of standard units of service. If these variations in quality were ignored, the true quantity of medical services would not be accurately measured. Of course, the price of standard units of service would not be constant if, as has frequently been alleged, doctors either discriminate in price according to wealth or derive psychic benefits from treating the poor. Given this type of variation, outlays would be positively correlated with price and hence would overstate the quantity of services purchased provided the elasticity of the MEC schedule were less than unity. But note that there is a factor at work that tends to counteract the effect of price discrimination. Since the average federal income tax rate rises with income, the value of tax deductions allowed for medical expenditures is greater for wealthier individuals.

The price of medical care might also vary across consumers because of the existence of health insurance. This would be the case if an individual's premium depended not on the size of his potential loss (medical outlays) in unfavorable states of the world and on his probability of incurring the loss but on the expected outlays and expected probability of a large group of persons. In this situation, the relevant price would be cP, where c is the fraction of medical expenditures not financed by insurance. If c were correlated with the independent variables in the demand curves for health and medical care, their coefficients would be biased. These biases would be mitigated to the extent that c does not vary greatly or to the extent that premiums are not entirely fixed.

Although the stock of health is difficult to define and measure empirically, a proxy for it is available in the NORC sample. Persons in the sample were asked whether their health status was, in general, poor, fair, good, or excellent. Their response to this question is utilized as an index of the amount of health capital they possess. This measure of H suffers from the defect that it depends on an individual's *subjective* evaluation of the state of his health: what one person considers to be excellent health may be viewed as good or only fair health by another. Moreover, it is not obvious how to quantify the four possible responses. That is, one must determine exactly how much more health capital a person in, say, excellent health has compared to someone in poor health.

Nothing can be done about the subjective nature of the health status variable, but it is possible to construct a particular scaling scheme. The procedure employed is based on two propositions. First, since the units of health capital are unknown, it seems reasonable to view the four quantities assigned to health status as measures of H in index number form. Thus, if $H = 1$ for people whose health status is poor, the three other quantities would express a person's stock relative to the stock of those in poor health. Second, the observed gross correlation between medical outlays and sick time is positive. It has already been indicated that this correlation reflects the positive relationship between medical care and the depreciation rate.

Using the second proposition, assume that the gross relation between the stock of health and medical expenditures is

$$H = aM^{-b}, a \text{ and } b > 0 \tag{4-11}$$

and let M_P, M_F, M_G, and M_E be mean outlays by people in poor, fair, good, and excellent health. Then to express the stock of health in index number form with $H_P = 1$, write $H_F/H_P = (M_P/M_F)^b$, etc. In the NORC sample, $M_P/M_F = 1.7$, $M_P/M_G = 2.3$, $M_P/M_E = 5.0$.[17] Thus, the health capital series is 1, 1.7, 2.3, and 5.0. It should be clear that a multiplicative

[17] These ratios pertain to whites in the labor force who reported positive sick time. See the end of this section and the beginning of Chapter V, Section 1, for the reasons why this group was used.

relation between H and M was selected to free the computed health series of units.[18]

Since the numerical magnitudes of health capital depend on medical expenditures, one might think at first that the coefficients of the stock demand curve would be related to those of the medical care demand curve. For example, if B_{XM} were the coefficient of variable X in the medical care demand curve, then equation (4-11) would seem to imply that the regression coefficient of $\ln H$ on X would be $-bB_{XM}$. This analysis, however, is not correct because equation (4-11) is not applied to individual observations. Instead, it is used to construct four quantities of H from data grouped by health status. Hence, the only purpose of this equation is to derive a health series in which increases in the stock of health reflect improvements in health status.[19] To emphasize this point and to show the effect of selecting different values for health status, two other sets of scales are employed in some of the regressions run in the next chapter These are $1 = $ poor, $2 = $ fair, $3 = $ good, $4 = $ excellent; and $0 = $ poor, $206 = $ fair, $290 = $ good, $411 = $ excellent. The first is an arbitrary set that has no relation to medical expenditures. The second is based on the *differences* between M_P and the outlays of those in the other three groups instead of on the ratios.

The remainder of this section discusses the independent variables that enter the demand curves for health and medical care. Age is simply given by the age of the individual. Education is the number of years of formal schooling completed by the head of the household. That is, if two or more members of a family are in the labor force, E is the same for each one. Since the head of the household is in most cases the husband, E is more accurately measured for males. Therefore, at one point in the empirical analysis, separate regressions are run for males and females. Moreover, to test the hypothesis that females might be more efficient producers of health than males (or vice versa), a sex dummy ($1 = $ female) is included in all regressions computed with persons of both sexes.

---

[18] If a linear relationship were used, then $H = a - bM$, and $H_F - H_P = b(M_P - M_F)$, etc. This series would not be free of units. Note also that the dependent variable in the stock demand curve should be $\ln H_j/H_P$ ($j = F, G, E$). Therefore, the use of $\ln M_j/M_P$ as the dependent variable would generate coefficients that would exceed, equal, or fall short of the true coefficients as b exceeds, equals, or falls short of 1. But because b is a constant, the t ratios associated with these coefficients would be unaffected.

[19] For some empirical evidence that the estimated regression coefficients in the demand curve for health capital are *not* linear transformations of the regression coefficients in the demand curve for medical care, see Chapter V, Tables 1 and 3.

A difficulty arises when education is used to measure human capital. The stock of human capital possessed by a person who has completed his formal education is not constant over the remainder of his life cycle. Instead, it tends to increase at first due to on-the-job training and then decrease due to depreciation. To the extent that age is correlated with human capital, its regression coefficient might reflect forces other than the depreciation rate. But since this correlation is positive during the early stages of the life cycle and negative during the later stages, its net effect on the age coefficient is not clear.

The wage rate variable is defined as follows. Let EA be actual earnings reported by a person and N be net earnings lost due to work-loss (gross earning lost minus disability insurance payments). Then $W = (52/WW)$ $(EA + N)$. Put differently, the relevant wage rate variable is the full-time annual equivalent of the weekly wage rate adjusted for variations in net earnings lost per work-loss week.[20]

The weekly wage can be written as

$$\frac{W}{52} = \frac{EA}{WW^*} \frac{WW^*}{WW} + \frac{N}{WLW} \frac{WLW}{WW},$$

where WW^* is the number of weeks actually worked, WLW is the number of work-loss weeks, and $WW = WW^* + WLW$. Note that if the weekly wage were not adjusted for variations in net earnings lost per work-loss week, a spurious negative relation would be created between the wage and sick time with the causality running from sick time to the wage instead of the other way around. This would occur if the wage were measured by EA/WW. In theory, the most desirable wage variable is the hourly wage rate, but unfortunately, hours of work per week were not available. To the extent that people with higher stocks of health work more hours per week than those with lower stocks, the causal relationship that goes from health to the wage has not been entirely eliminated. Note also that with all other variables held constant, a reduction in net earnings lost per work-loss week, N/WLW, would reduce $W/52$. Hence, the actual wage rate used in the regression analysis takes some account of the effect of informal sick leave arrangements and disability insurance on the value of the marginal product of health capital.[21]

[20] Since ln W is the dependent variable in all regressions, its coefficient would be the same whether or not the weekly wage rate were multiplied by 52.

[21] A more complete discussion of this point appears in the last subsection of Chapter V, Section 1. There I indicate why it would be inappropriate to use N/WLW as an index of the benefits from reducing sick time.

As in most cross-sectional studies, the NORC sample contains data on income but not wealth. Hence, the former is used as a proxy variable for the latter. Regardless of whether wealth or income measures a person's command over real resources, since a family pools its resources, family wealth or family income (Y) is the appropriate variable to enter in the demand functions.[22] This follows even though the dependent variables— H, $WLD1$, RAD, and M—pertain to a particular individual in a given family.

To free family income of transitory components associated with variations in weeks worked and net earnings lost, it must be adjusted in the manner that is employed to adjust earnings. Certain difficulties arise here because the number of wage earners is not the same in every family. Since labor force participation of married women is inversely related to husband's income, families with one wage earner might have more full income (defined as full potential family earnings plus family property income) but less reported income than families with two wage earners. To deal with this problem, four concepts of family income are utilized: $Y1$, $Y2$, $Y3$, and $Y4$. The first two income variables are partially adjusted for variations in weeks worked, the third is fully adjusted, and the fourth is unadjusted. These variables are defined as follows. Let V be family property income, n be the number of members in a given family who are in the labor force, and the subscript 1 identify the member of the family who worked the most number of weeks in 1963. Then

$$Y1 = V + (52/WW_1)(EA_1 + N_1)$$

$$Y2 = Y1 + \sum_{j=2}^{n} (EA_j + N_j)$$

$$Y3 = V + \sum_{j=1}^{n} (52/WW_j)(EA_j + N_j)$$

$$Y4 = V + \sum_{j=1}^{n} (EA_j + N_j).$$

Obviously, $Y1 = Y2 = Y3$ for families with only one wage earner. In addition, note that $Y4$ does take account of net earnings lost by all family members.

The variables just described place an upper and lower limit on potential family income. The upper limit is given by $Y3$, the lower limit

[22] As I point out later, family income per capita might be used. In any case, one would not want to simply enter the income reported by a given family member.

by $Y1$ or $Y4$, and a value that lies between these two extremes by $Y2$.[23] Hopefully, the income elasticities computed with these four variables will bracket the true parameter.[24]

The regression equations fitted to the NORC data contain family income, an individual's weekly wage rate, and his level of education as independent variables. Since Y, W, and E are all positively correlated, one might be puzzled at first by the interpretation to be given to the procedure of parceling out the separate effects of each via the multiple regression technique. Variations in property income could explain why two people with different full-time earnings have the same income. But how could two persons with the same amount of education have different wage rates when it is by this time well-accepted that an increase in education raises market productivity? Robert Michael has considered this question and has concluded that there are a variety of possible answers: "different relative degrees of labor shortage or abundance in different occupations, different degrees of monopoly power or of union strength, different innate ability, ... different amounts of on-the-job training ... or other forms of human capital, [and] luck."[25] Thus, it is possible at a conceptual level to raise W, Y, or E with the other two fixed. Of course, if these variables were subject to errors of measurement, their coefficients would be biased; the sources and directions of these biases are discussed in Appendix D, Section 2.

The last explanatory variable in the demand functions is family size (FS). This variable is included in the regressions for two reasons. First, the number of children in a family and the health stocks of its adult members might be complements. This is a plausible hypothesis because the lower the amount of sick time the more time there is available for childrearing activities. Second, since the dependent variables pertain to individuals and not families, per capita income might be a more appropriate measure of command over real resources than family income. This is easily accomplished if family income and family size enter the regressions.[26]

[23] Although $Y1$ exceeds $Y4$ for one wage earner families, the mean of $Y4$ exceeds that of $Y1$ in the NORC sample.

[24] Since income is used as an empirical proxy for wealth, the term income elasticity is substituted for wealth elasticity from now on.

[25] *The Effect of Education on Efficiency in Consumption*, New York, NBER, Occasional Paper 116, 1972, p. 29.

[26] If $\ln H = B_{W/P_0} \ln Y/FS + B_{P_0} \ln FS$ then $\ln H = B_{W/P_0} \ln Y + (B_{P_0} - B_{W/P_0}) \ln FS$ Hence, the use of family income instead of per capita income alters the coefficient of family size alone.

One final comment on the regression analysis is in order. Whites in the NORC sample reported more sick days than nonwhites, which contradicts data in the U.S. National Health Survey.[27] Since there were few nonwhites in the sample, it was felt that the data for them might be unreliable. Consequently, it was decided to restrict the analysis to whites in the labor force. The sample size of this group is 1,770.

3. GLOSSARY

α_1 Share of medical care in total cost of gross investment or elasticity of gross investment with respect to medical care
RAD   Restricted-activity days
WLD   Work-loss days
WW   Weeks worked
*WLD*1   Work-loss days adjusted for variations in weeks worked
EA   Earnings
N   Net earnings lost due to work-loss
*Y*1, *Y*2,
*Y*3, *Y*4   Various measures of family income
FS   Family size

[27] See Geraldine A. Gleeson and Elijah L. White, "Disability and Medical Care Among Whites and Nonwhites in the United States," *Health, Education, and Welfare Indicators* (October 1965). The U.S. National Health Survey is a continuing probability sample that contains approximately 40,000 households. It was not used in this study because data from it are available only at a fairly aggregate level.

V

EMPIRICAL RESULTS:
THE NORC SAMPLE

This chapter presents empirical estimates of demand curves for health and medical care and gross investment production functions. The first part of the chapter contains the analysis performed with whites in the labor force who reported positive sick time in 1963. This analysis is emphasized because of the 1,770 persons in the labor force, 558 had some sick days in 1963 and 1,212 had no sick days. Since the characteristics of these two groups are very similar, it is difficult to explain the behavior of the latter. Put differently, the two groups essentially represent "two different samples," and problems arise when the data are pooled. The second part discusses these difficulties and also shows how the results are affected by excluding females from the regressions.

1. WHITES WITH POSITIVE SICK TIME

Demand Curves for Health and Medical Care

Tables 1, 2, and 3 present alternative estimates of health stock, health flow, and medical care demand curves. Five demand curves appear for

TABLE 1

Stock Demand for Health by Whites with Positive Sick Time

$(N = 558)$

Income Measure	ln Y	ln W	E	i	Sex	ln FS	$\bar{R}^2$
$Y1$	.004	.127	.025	−.009	−.092	−.018	.171
	(.09)	(2.41)	(4.05)	(−6.23)	(−1.90)	(−.45)	
$Y2$	.049	.098	.025	−.009	−.108	−.027	.172
	(.99)	(2.01)	(4.12)	(−6.32)	(−2.15)	(−.69)	
$Y4$	.063	.090	.025	−.009	−.112	−.033	.174
	(1.41)	(1.95)	(4.11)	(−6.36)	(−2.26)	(−.82)	
$Y4$[a]	.117		.029	−.009	−.159	−.049	.170
	(3.36)		(5.09)	(−6.25)	(−3.64)	(−1.26)	
Y omitted		.130	.025	−.009	−.091	−.017	.172
		(3.63)	(4.06)	(−6.26)	(−1.93)	(−.45)	

NOTE: N indicates the sample size, t ratios are in parentheses, and intercepts are not shown. For definitions of the three income variables, see Chapter IV, Section 2.

[a] In this regression, the wage rate is excluded.

TABLE 2
Flow Demand for Health by Whites with Positive Sick Time

Income Measure	ln Y	ln W	E	i	Sex	ln FS	$\bar{R}^2$
			$TL = WLD1$				
$Y1$	−.280	.554	.046	−.006	.010	.251	.087
	(−2.03)	(4.01)	(2.87)	(−1.67)	(.08)	(2.46)	
$Y2$	−.221	.497	.044	−.007	.033	.261	.085
	(−1.72)	(3.88)	(2.74)	(−1.75)	(.25)	(2.51)	
$Y4$	−.031	.367	.046	−.007	−.032	.222	.080
	(−.26)	(3.04)	(2.86)	(−1.86)	(−.25)	(2.12)	
$Y4^a$	.193		.063	−.007	−.223	.155	.067
	(2.08)		(4.14)	(−1.68)	(−1.93)	(1.51)	
Y omitted		.349	.046	−.007	−.043	.214	.082
		(3.69)	(2.87)	(−1.89)	(−.34)	(2.13)	
			$TL = RAD$				
$Y1$	−.282	.392	.046	−.009	−.072	.226	.063
	(−1.97)	(2.74)	(2.77)	(−2.17)	(−.54)	(2.15)	
$Y2$	−.248	.352	.044	−.009	−.040	.242	.062
	(−1.85)	(2.65)	(2.64)	(−2.23)	(−.30)	(2.25)	
$Y4$	−.147	.280	.046	−.009	−.076	.226	.058
	(−1.21)	(2.33)	(2.73)	(−2.28)	(−.56)	(2.09)	
$Y4^a$	.023		.058	−.009	−.222	.176	.052
	(.24)		(3.73)	(−2.15)	(−1.86)	(1.65)	
Y omitted		.186	.046	−.010	−.125	.190	.058
		(1.89)	(2.77)	(−2.38)	(−.97)	(1.82)	

NOTE: See the notes to Table 1.

each of the four dependent variables—ln H, − ln $WLD1$, − ln RAD, and ln M.[1] In the first three regressions, family income equals $Y1$, $Y2$, or $Y4$. The fourth regression shows how the coefficients are affected if income is measured by $Y4$ and the wage rate is excluded. The last regression includes the wage but leaves out income.

As a guide to interpreting these regressions, Table 4 shows the means and coefficients of variation of the four endogenous variables. Since individuals are the units of observation, the coefficients of variation are

[1] Since 2.4 percent of the sample reported no medical outlays, M, and not its natural logarithm, is the dependent variable in Table 3. All regression coefficients were converted to elasticities or percentage changes at the mean by multiplying by $1/\bar{M}$. These elasticities or percentage changes are presented in Table 3.

TABLE 3

Demand for Medical Care by Whites with Positive Sick Time

Income Measure	ln Y	ln W	E	i	Sex	ln FS	$\bar{R}^2$
Y1	.701	−.170	.009	.016	.597	−.122	.063
	(3.36)	(−.81)	(.35)	(2.66)	(3.10)	(−.79)	
Y2	.754	−.162	.015	.016	.473	−.190	.069
	(3.87)	(−.84)	(.62)	(2.71)	(2.37)	(−1.21)	
Y4	.695	−.105	.012	.016	.499	−.204	.070
	(3.92)	(−.57)	(.47)	(2.72)	(2.54)	(−1.29)	
Y4^a	.632		.007	.016	.554	−.185	.071
	(4.57)		(.29)	(2.70)	(3.21)	(−1.20)	
Y omitted		.343	.008	.018	.730	−.031	.046
		(2.38)	(.33)	(3.00)	(3.83)	(−.20)	

NOTE: See the notes to Table 1.

TABLE 4

Means and Coefficients of Variation,
Endogenous Variables

Variable	Mean	Coefficient of Variation (percent)
H^a	3.1	47.0
$WLD1^b$	16.6 days	194.1
RAD	16.3 days	211.4
M	$208.2	179.7

^{a} The frequency distribution of health status is as follows: excellent, 35.7 percent of sample; good, 41.8 percent; fair, 17.9 percent; poor, 4.7 percent.

^{b} The mean of WLD1 exceeds the mean of RAD because reported work-loss was multiplied by 52/WW—a number that is equal to or greater than unity.

extremely large. This explains why the coefficients of multiple determination ($\bar{R}^2$) are relatively low.[2] The correlation coefficient between WLD1 and RAD is .835, which indicates the close relation between these two measures of sick days.

[2] J. S. Cramer has shown that in the absence of errors of measurement, grouping the data by the independent variables would *raise* the R^2, *reduce* the t ratios associated with regression coefficients, and *have no effect* on the expected value of the estimate of the residual variance. See "Efficient Grouping, Regression and Correlation in Engel Curve Analysis," *Journal of the American Statistical Association*, 59, No. 5 (March 1964).

Since the coefficients of the investment model depend on the elasticity of the MEC schedule, it is helpful to estimate ε. This parameter can be computed from the production function of healthy days given by

$$h = 365 - BH^{-C},$$

or

$$-\ln TL = -\ln B + C \ln H,$$

since it has been shown that $\varepsilon = 1/(1 + C)$. Using $-\ln WLD1$ and $-\ln RAD$ as alternative proxies for $-\ln TL$, I obtained the following two regressions:

$$-\ln WLD1 = .854 \ln H$$
$$(8.58) \qquad\qquad \varepsilon = .54$$
$$-\ln RAD = .955 \ln H$$
$$(9.49) \qquad\qquad \varepsilon = .51$$

In neither case is the regression coefficient significantly different from one at the .05 level of confidence on a two tail test. Therefore, it is concluded that the best estimate of ε is .5.

Table 5 shows the effects of selecting alternative sets of scales for health status on the stock demand curve. Series A is the one stressed in

TABLE 5
Stock Demand Curves, Alternative Health Capital Series

ln Y4	ln W	E	i	Sex	ln FS	$\bar{R}^2$
			Series A[a]			
.171	.252	.067	−.028	−.360	−.096	.153
(1.25)	(1.78)	(3.59)	(−6.09)	(−2.37)	(−.79)	
			Series B[a]			
.094	.177	.049	−.017	−.166	−.034	.189
(1.20)	(2.21)	(4.59)	(−6.54)	(−1.92)	(−.49)	
			Series C[a]			
14.927	19.466	5.789	−1.927	−20.321	−7.253	.181
(1.60)	(2.02)	(4.52)	(−6.23)	(−1.96)	(−.87)	

[a] See the text for definition.

Chapter IV and used in Table 1: 1 = poor, 1.7 = fair, 2.3 = good, 5.0 = excellent. In Series B, the four values of health status are 1 = poor, 2 = fair, 3 = good, 4 = excellent; and in Series C, these four values are 0 = poor, 206 = fair, 290 = good, 411 = excellent.[3] Since health capital can equal zero in the last series, H, and not ln H, is the dependent variable in all three regressions. Although the magnitudes of the regression coefficients vary with the series employed, their signs do not vary, and their t ratios are fairly insensitive.[4] These findings should strengthen our confidence in the results obtained with Series A. This series, like the theoretical index, is free of units. Therefore, there is some justification for the magnitudes of its regression coefficients.

A comparison of the results in Tables 1 and 3 reveals that although medical outlays were used to scale health capital, the estimated regression coefficients in the health stock demand curve are not linear transformations of the regression coefficients in the medical care demand curve. For example, the coefficient of education in the health stock demand curve is .025 with a t ratio of approximately 4. The corresponding coefficient in the medical care demand curve is approximately .010 with a t ratio of approximately .5.

The estimated demand parameters of age, education, the wage rate, family income, sex, and family size are now discussed in detail. The regression coefficients of age are negative in the health stock and health flow demand curves, while the regression coefficient is positive in the medical care demand curve. These signs are exactly what would be expected if depreciation rates rose with age and if the elasticity of the MEC schedule were less than unity. All regression coefficients are significant at the .05 level of confidence on a one-tail test, and their magnitudes are independent of the family income variable employed. The results indicate that health capital falls over the life cycle at a continuously compounded rate of .9 percent per year. The rates of increase in restricted-activity days, work-loss days, and medical outlays are .9, .7, and 1.6 percent per year, respectively.

The estimates of ε and $\tilde{H}$ can be used to compute $\tilde{\delta}$, the continuously compounded rate of increase in the depreciation rate over the life cycle. The age parameter in the stock demand curve is $-s_i\tilde{\delta}\varepsilon = .009$. Since $\varepsilon = .5$, one can solve for $\tilde{\delta}$ by assigning arbitrary values to s_i, the share

---

[3] See Chapter IV, Section 2, for a discussion of these three series.

[4] These conclusions hold when $Y1$ or $Y2$ replaces $Y4$ as the measure of family income.

of depreciation in the cost of health capital. For values of s_i that range from .25 to 1, the estimates of $\tilde{\delta}$ are:[5]

s_i	$\tilde{\delta}$
.25	7.2%
.50	3.6
.75	2.4
1.00	1.8

Since s_i rises with age, $\tilde{\delta}$ is unlikely to be as large as 7.2 percent. Perhaps the best estimate is an average of the last two rates or 2.1 percent.

Suppose none of the reduction in health capital associated with a given increase in the rate of depreciation were offset by an increase in gross investment. Then the number of periods it would take for a certain percentage of a person's initial stock of health to depreciate could be calculated.[6] With $\tilde{\delta} = 2.1$ percent, 70 percent of the initial stock would depreciate by age 58, 80 percent by age 77, and 90 percent by age 96. In fact, medical outlays rise over the life cycle so that these ages understate the time that must elapse before the stock of health falls to specified levels. If, for example, the ratio of the death stock to the initial stock were .3, individuals would not die at age 58. Instead, because the demand for health is relatively inelastic, they would have an incentive to postpone death by investing more at later than at earlier ages.

Whether health is measured by H, $-WLD1$, or $-RAD$, the regression coefficient of education is positive and statistically significant at conventional levels. It is seen that the continuously compounded rate of growth in health capital for a one year increase in the level of formal schooling is 2.5 percent. The rates of decrease in the number of work-loss days and the number of restricted-activity days are both equal to 4.6 percent. These results imply that an increase in education raises the marginal products of the direct inputs in the gross investment production function, lowers marginal cost, and shifts the MEC schedule to the right. Therefore, the demand for health increases. Since there is reason to believe the elasticity of the MEC schedule is less than unity, education should be

---

[5] Since $\tilde{H}$ equals $\widehat{RAD}$ and is only slightly greater than $\widehat{WLD1}$, the calculations of $\tilde{\delta}$ would not be affected if the flow parameters were utilized. Note that the age-health profile is concave to the origin for $s_i < 1$, which suggests that the square of age should be added to the set of independent variables. Attempts to do this were not successful because age and age squared are extremely highly correlated.

[6] If none of the increase in $\tilde{\delta}$ were offset, then $H_i = H_1 \exp(-\tilde{\delta}i)$. Given $\tilde{\delta}$, one can find the age at which H_i/H_1 equals, for example, .1.

negatively correlated with medical expenditures. In fact, the regression coefficient is positive but not significant.

The education parameter in the health demand curve is given by $r_H \varepsilon$, where r_H is the percentage improvement in health productivity per unit increase in E or the percentage reduction in marginal cost. Since $\varepsilon = .5$, the stock coefficient suggests r_H equals 5.0 percent, and the flow coefficient suggests it equals 9.2 percent.[7] An average of these two estimates indicates that the marginal cost of producing gross additions to health capital is roughly 7.1 percent lower for consumers with, say, eleven years of formal schooling compared to those with ten years.

In accordance with the a priori notion that an increase in the wage rate raises the monetary return and hence the rate of return on an investment in health, the wage is positively related to the stock of health and the number of healthy days. All wage elasticities of health are statistically significant but tend to vary with the measure of family income employed. Therefore, the first column of Table 6 shows the average of, for instance, the stock elasticities obtained with the three family income variables. Mean wage elasticities of H, $-WLD1$, and $-RAD$ are .105, .471, and .341, respectively. The large magnitudes of the flow elasticities are more consistent with the investment model than with the consumption model.[8]

TABLE 6

Average Wage, Income, and Family Size Elasticities

Dependent Variable	Average Wage Elasticity	Average Income Elasticity	Average Family Size Elasticity
ln H	.105	.039	.013
$-$ln $WLD1$	.471	$-$.177	.067
$-$ln RAD	.341	$-$.226	.006
ln M	$-$.146	.717	.545

[7] Since the best estimate of C is unity, stock and flow regression coefficients of a given variable should be equal. Although the age coefficients are very similar, the flow coefficient of education is almost twice as large as the stock coefficient. This accounts for the variation in the estimate of r_H.

[8] To the extent that people must be paid higher than average wages to enter occupations or industries that are detrimental to health, wage elasticity estimates are biased *downward*. In addition, it should be realized that the analysis is limited to members of the labor force. Thus, any statements about the superiority of the investment model relative to the consumption model pertain to this group alone.

An upward shift in the wage rate should not only increase health but also medical care. Unfortunately, the wage elasticity of medical care is negative but not significant.

The wage elasticity of health equals $(1 - K)\varepsilon$, where K is the fraction of the total cost of gross investment accounted for by time. According to the stock elasticity estimate, K equals .79, and according to the flow elasticity, it equals .19.[9] The mean of these two time shares is .49. If the average time intensity of nonmarket production equaled .5, gross investment in health would be neither a goods-intensive activity nor a time-intensive activity. Of course, this is merely a tentative conclusion because the average time intensity is unknown and because the estimate of K has a large variance.

It should be noted that the effects of measurement errors may explain why education and the wage rate have the "wrong signs" in the demand curve for medical care.[10] Appendix D, Section 2, indicates that regression coefficients are influenced by measurement error for two reasons. First, the wage rate is likely to contain random errors of observation. Second, with education held constant, the wage rate is probably positively correlated with other determinants of nonmarket efficiency, such as innate ability. Under certain conditions, it can be shown that these two forces bias the estimated wage elasticity of health in *opposite* directions; measurement error biases it downward, ability biases it upward, and the net effect is not clear. Similarly, the education coefficient in the health demand curve is biased in opposite directions. On the other hand, the two sources of bias operate in the *same* direction on any given coefficient in the demand curve for medical care. In particular, they bias the wage elasticity downward and the education coefficient upward.[11]

---

[9] The calculation of K from the flow parameters uses an average of the wage elasticities of $-WLD1$ and $-RAD$.

[10] Jacob Mincer points out that the observed effects of the wage rate and education on medical outlays can also be explained by assuming that the stock of health is one determinant of the wage rate. Mincer postulates that with the wage fixed, an increase in education may be accompanied by a decrease in health and other forms of human capital. Since a reduction in health is likely to increase medical outlays, the education coefficient would be biased upward. The difficulty with this explanation is that it tends to be contradicted by the health demand curve estimates. With the wage constant, healthy time and the index of health capital are positively related to education.

[11] Suppose the two biases exactly offset each other in the health demand curve. Then the expected value of any regression coefficient would be an unbiased estimate of the corresponding population parameter. In this situation, one can, for example, use the wage elasticity of health to solve for the wage elasticity of medical care. He can then force the

Before the effects of family income are summarized, recall that $Y1$ and $Y2$ are partially adjusted for variations in weeks worked, while $Y4$ is not adjusted. The relationship between each of these three income variables and the stock of health is positive but not significant at conventional levels. On the other hand, income effects are *negative* in the flow demand curves. When $Y1$ or $Y2$ enters the regressions, flow income elasticities are statistically significant. The elasticities are not significant when $Y4$ enters and are much smaller in absolute value. In contrast to the negative or weak positive health income elasticities, the income elasticities of medical care are all positive and very significant.

To check the validity of the income elasticity estimates, these coefficients were recomputed after excluding members of "atypical families" —those with three or more wage earners—from the sample. In the regressions run with persons from families with one or two wage earners, family income fully adjusted for variations in weeks worked by all members ($Y3$) was added to the set of income proxies. Income elasticities for this group are as follows:[12]

Income Measure	ln H	$-$ ln $WLD1$	$-$ ln RAD	ln M
$Y1$	$-.005$	$-.285$	$-.288$	.722
$Y2$	.041	$-.238$	$-.251$	.752
$Y3$	.032	$-.240$	$-.213$	.611
$Y4$	.057	$-.040$	$-.149$	.693
Average elasticity	.031	$-.201$	$-.225$	.695

The average income elasticities are almost identical to those for all whites with positive sick time, which are given by column 2 of Table 6. Moreover, $Y3$ elasticities are in most cases very similar to $Y2$ elasticities.

It should be noted that income has a negative effect on the number of healthy days and a positive but weak effect on the amount of health capital only if the wage rate is held constant. When the wage is left out of the regressions, health income elasticities are positive and, with the exception of the RAD elasticity, statistically significant. The simple

---

wage coefficient to assume its proper value in the demand curve for medical care and see how the estimates of the other coefficients in this function are affected. For some a priori estimates along these lines, see Appendix E, Section 1.

[12] The sample size is 542. The coefficients of the other exogenous variables are quite similar to those in Tables 1, 2, and 3.

correlation coefficients between ln W and ln $Y1$, ln $Y2$, and ln $Y4$ are .754, .645, and .606, respectively. Hence, health income elasticities are seriously biased by the omission of the wage rate.[13]

The consumption model predicts a positive correlation between health and income, while the investment model predicts a zero correlation. This raises the question: How should one interpret the negative income elasticity of healthy days? Some readers may say that this finding is artificial, for if the wage rate is one of the independent variables, it is not meaningful to include income as an additional explanatory variable. For the benefit of these readers, Tables 1, 2, and 3 reveal that gross wage elasticities of health—elasticities obtained when family income is omitted from the regressions—always exceed gross income elasticities. Furthermore, the gross wage elasticity of medical care is positive and significant, as the investment model would predict. I would argue, however, that it is meaningful to include both family income and the wage in the regressions. These variables are not so highly correlated that the results are dominated by multicollinearity. In addition, the gross wage elasticity of medical care is much smaller than the gross income elasticity (.343 compared with .632). This suggests that income has an effect in the model that is at least partly independent of the wage effect.

Given that my procedure is valid, does the negative income elasticity of healthy days imply health is an inferior commodity? If the consumption aspects of health were at all relevant, then a literal interpretation of the income coefficient would suggest that this is in fact the case. It is possible, however, to account for the negative income elasticity of health without assuming it is an inferior commodity. The explanation offered in the next chapter stresses that medical care is not the only market input in the gross investment production function. Instead, inputs such as diet, exercise, recreation goods, alcohol, cigarettes, and rich food are also relevant. The last three inputs have *negative* marginal products, and if their income elasticities exceeded the income elasticities of the beneficial inputs, the shadow price of health would be positively correlated with

[13] For a similar conclusion, see Morris Silver, "An Economic Analysis of Variations in Medical Expenses and Work-Loss Rates," in Herbert E. Klarman (ed.), *Empirical Studies in Health Economics*, Baltimore, 1970, and reprinted as Chapter 6 in Victor R. Fuchs (ed.), *Essays in the Economics of Health and Medical Care*, New York, NBER, 1972. Although Silver's interpretation of the negative health elasticity differs from the one I present in Chapter VI, he should be credited for stressing the importance of holding the wage constant. It should also be indicated that the partial correlation between ln Y and ln W is relevant in an examination of "omitted variable bias." But in the NORC sample, this correlation coefficient is approximately equal to the simple correlation.

income. This appears to be a promising explanation because it can also account for the positive correlation between medical care and income. That is, it can show the conditions under which persons with higher incomes would simultaneously reduce their demand for health and increase their demand for medical care.

The role of the sex dummy variable (1 = female) in the health demand curves is somewhat ambiguous. Females have significantly smaller stocks of health than males, more restricted-activity days, but fewer work-loss days except when income is measured by $Y4$. In the demand curve for medical care, the coefficient of the sex dummy indicates that outlays by women are approximately 50 percent higher than outlays by men. Although these results are generally consistent with the hypothesis that males are more efficient producers of health than females, they are also undoubtedly related to childbearing.

Column 3 of Table 6 gives average family size elasticities of health and medical care. These elasticities are computed by summing the actual coefficients of $\ln Y$ and $\ln FS$ and are the coefficients that would be obtained if command over resources were measured by per capita income. Family size is positively correlated with each of the three indexes of health and also with medical care. One interpretation of these correlations is that the number of children in a family and the health levels of its adult members are complements.

The Gross Investment Production Function

Table 7 presents ordinary least squares and two-stage least squares estimates of gross investment production functions. In the ordinary least squares regressions, the elasticities of the three measures of health with respect to medical services are all *negative*, which reflects the strong positive relation between medical care and the depreciation rate. The two-stage regressions employ values of M predicted from its demand curve.[14] It is seen that when income is excluded from the second stage, the elasticities of H and $-WLD1$ with respect to M are both positive and approximately equal to .2, while the elasticity of $-RAD$ is negative. If income is included as a proxy for other market inputs in the production function, the elasticity of H is reduced to .1. On the other hand, the elasticities of $-WLD1$ and $-RAD$ rise to .5 and .3. Income itself is negatively related to $-WLD1$ and $-RAD$ but positively related to H.

[14] The prediction equation uses per capita income and sets the family size coefficient equal to .491. Per capita income is measured by $Y4/FS$ because this variable gives the medical care demand curve with the highest $\bar{R}^2$.

TABLE 7

Gross Investment Production Functions of Whites with Positive Sick Time

Dependent Variable	ln M	E	i	Sex	ln $Y4/FS$	$\bar{R}^2$
			Two-Stage Least Squares			
ln H	.170	.029	−.012	−.248		.168
	(3.13)	(4.93)	(−6.52)	(−4.78)		
ln H	.098	.029	−.011	−.219	.044	.168
	(.97)	(4.93)	(−5.21)	(−3.48)	(.84)	
−ln $WLD1$	.224	.060	−.012	−.418		.059
	(1.55)	(3.87)	(−2.41)	(−3.02)		
−ln $WLD1$	.545	.060	−.015	−.550	−.198	.060
	(2.01)	(3.88)	(−2.79)	(−3.29)	(−1.40)	
−ln RAD	−.024	.057	−.010	−.269		.048
	(−.16)	(3.58)	(−1.95)	(−1.89)		
−ln RAD	.275	.057	−.013	−.391	−.184	.049
	(.99)	(3.59)	(−2.32)	(−2.28)	(−1.27)	
			Ordinary Least Squares			
ln H	−.060	.036	−.007	−.117		.203
	(−5.84)	(6.73)	(−5.02)	(−2.83)		
ln H	−.068	.030	−.008	−.143	.117	.226
	(−6.54)	(5.47)	(−5.91)	(−3.49)	(4.33)	
−ln $WLD1$	−.294	.007	−.001	−.124		.241
	(−11.66)	(5.85)	(−.33)	(−1.23)		
−ln $WLDI$	−.304	.068	−.003	−.163	.175	.249
	(−11.98)	(4.99)	(−.89)	(−1.61)	(2.56)	
−ln RAD	−.334	.067	−.003	−.093		.277
	(−13.24)	(5.11)	(−.98)	(−.93)		
−ln RAD	−.339	.063	−.004	−.112	.085	.278
	(−13.28)	(4.60)	(−1.23)	(−1.11)	(1.24)	

Although it is encouraging that the utilization of two-stage least squares generates positive medical care elasticities of health, these results should be interpreted with *extreme* caution. This follows because they are very sensitive to the particular set of variables excluded from the second stage (FS and W or FS, W, and $Y4/FS$). Moreover, the production function coefficients of education and age should be similar to the estimates of r_H and $\tilde{\delta}$ previously computed. Instead, they are almost identical to the actual demand curve coefficients. For these reasons, it is better to emphasize the demand curves that were fitted to the data than to emphasize the production function.

The Role of Disability Insurance

Table 8 introduces two disability insurance dummy variables into the demand curves for health and medical care. The members of the NORC sample who reported positive sick time were not asked whether they were potentially eligible for disability insurance benefits. Instead, only those who had positive gross earnings lost due to work-loss were asked if they received disability benefits. Of the 558 persons who had positive sick time, 285 had no gross earnings lost, 203 had positive gross earnings lost but did not receive disability payments, and 70 received such payments. To compare these three classes, two dummy variables, *Gross* and *Dis*, are used. They are coded as follows:

Class	Gross	Dis
No gross earning lost	0	1
Disability insurance	1	1
No disability insurance	1	0

In this form, the regression coefficient of *Gross* compares those with no gross earnings lost to those with disability benefits, the coefficient of *Dis* compares those who received benefits to those who did not, and the difference between the two coefficients compares those with no earnings lost to those with no insurance benefits.

The regressions in Table 8 reveal that persons who receive disability benefits had smaller stocks of health, more sick days, and higher medical outlays relative to persons with no benefits and relative to persons with no earnings lost.[15] The regressions also reveal that individuals with no gross earnings lost had larger quantities of health capital, fewer sick days, and smaller medical outlays compared to individuals with gross earnings lost but no disability benefits. Moreover, the coefficients of education in the health demand curves are the ones that are most affected by the introduction of the two dummies. Tables 1 and 2 show these coefficients are very significant when *Dis* and *Gross* are excluded from the regressions. If the dummies are held constant, the stock coefficient of education falls from .025 to .018, and the flow coefficients become insignificant. The coefficients of the other independent variables do not depart radically from those previously obtained.

As shown by the *t* ratio of *Dis* or *Gross*, the partial correlation between either of these two variables and sick time is larger than the partial

[15] The income variable in these regressions is $Y4$. The conclusions reached in the text are not altered when the other income variables are employed

TABLE 8

Demand Curves with Dummies Included for Disability Insurance and Gross Earnings Lost

Dependent Variable	ln Y4	ln W	E	i	Sex	ln FS	Dis	Gross	$\bar{R}^2$
ln H	.053	.086	.018	−.010	−.104	−.037	−.032	−.170	.192
	(1.29)	(1.90)	(2.85)	(−6.83)	(−2.11)	(−.94)	(−.54)	(−2.87)	
−ln WLD1	−.047	.349	.005	−.011	.008	.173	−1.009	−1.561	.245
	(−.44)	(3.18)	(.34)	(−3.18)	(.07)	(1.82)	(−6.96)	(−10.90)	
−ln RAD	−.160	.261	.005	−.013	−.036	.176	−1.058	−1.596	.221
	(−1.44)	(2.28)	(.30)	(−3.60)	(−.29)	(1.78)	(−7.02)	(−10.72)	
ln M	.698	−.086	.051	.021	.462	−.149	1.205	1.675	.151
	(4.11)	(−.49)	(2.11)	(3.54)	(2.45)	(−.99)	(5.23)	(7.37)	

correlation between sick time and any one of the basic exogenous variables in the model. Does this mean that *Dis* and *Gross* are the major determinants of sick time and that the education effects previously observed are spurious? In my judgment, this is not the case, for I would question the usefulness of holding *Dis* and *Gross* constant. Two factors suggest that the causal relationship runs not from these two variables to sick days but vice versa. In the first place, most informal sick leave arrangements allow employees a certain number of sick days before they begin to lose wages. In the second place, disability insurance plans typically begin to pay benefits only after the recipient has experienced a certain minimum number of sick days. For both these reasons, one would expect that the more sick days a respondent reported, the greater the likelihood that he lost earnings and received disability insurance benefits. This implies that the proper way to assess the impact of sick leave and disability plans on sick days would be to ask all individuals whether they are *potentially* eligible for the benefits provided by these plans. Since the NORC sample was not structured in this manner, the two dummies are, at least in part, proxy variables for sick time.

Additional considerations indicate that the education effects estimated in Tables 1 and 2 are the relevant ones. If an increase in education shifts the MEC schedule to the right, it would simultaneously increase the demand for healthy days and reduce observed gross earnings lost. In fact, *Gross* and *E* are strongly negatively correlated ($r = -.328$).[16] Since *Gross* is negatively correlated with $-\ln WLD1$, the regression coefficient of *E* is greatly increased when *Gross* is omitted. The simultaneous determination of earnings lost and sick days by education implies that one should not hold *Gross* constant in estimating the relationship between $-\ln WLD1$ and *E*.

Even if it is assumed that individuals are partially or fully compensated for their loss in market earnings due to illness, the general properties of my model are still valid. Persons would still have an incentive to demand health capital in order to reduce the time they lose from nonmarket activities and the disutility of illness. In addition, what may be termed "the inconvenience costs of illness" are positively correlated with the wage rate. That is, the complexity of a particular job and the amount of responsibility it entails certainly are positively related to the wage. Thus, when an individual with a high wage rate becomes ill, tasks that only he can perform accumulate. These increase the intensity of his work load

[16] The absolute value of this correlation coefficient is larger than that between *Gross* and any of the other independent variables

and give him an incentive to avoid illness by demanding more health capital.

Once disability insurance and sick leave arrangements are introduced, the value of the marginal product of health capital might not equal WG, but it would surely not equal zero. In the NORC sample, net earnings lost per work-loss day are positively correlated with the number of work-loss days ($r = .102$). Suppose the total loss in earnings due to work-loss is given by WTL, where W equals net earnings lost per day instead of the wage rate. Then the value of the marginal product of health capital would be $W(1 + 1/e_{TL})G$, where e_{TL} is the elasticity of the average loss with respect to sick days. Since this elasticity is positive, the marginal loss $W(1 + 1/e_{TL})$, exceeds the average loss. Therefore, the marginal rate of return on an investment in health might be substantial even if the average daily loss is small.[17]

The behavior of the average loss might explain why many educated persons report no gross earnings lost due to work-loss. Chapter II indicated that if health capital is viewed as a form of self-protection against uncertainty, the rate of return might equal zero in relatively desirable states of the world. Since the more educated have higher rates of return on a given stock of health than the less educated, they would have the greatest incentive to drive the rate of return to zero in relatively desirable states. Suppose individuals suffered no loss in earnings unless their sick time exceeded some maximum quantity TL^*. Then consumers with high levels of formal schooling could drive their rates of return to zero by holding enough health capital to make the number of sick days they experience less than TL^*.

2. SUPPLEMENTARY RESULTS

All Whites in the Labor Force

Table 9 presents health and medical care demand curves for all whites in the labor force. The income variable in these regressions is $Y4$.[18] Since persons with no sick days are included in these regressions, the

[17] If the average daily loss replaces the wage variable in the regressions, a simultaneous equations problem arises because the daily loss depends on sick time. By employing the wage as an index of the potential benefits from reducing sick time, this problem is avoided. Earlier it was shown that the weekly wage variable is positively correlated with net earnings lost per day. Therefore, it does take some account of the effect of informal sick leave arrangements and disability insurance on the value of the marginal product of health capital.

[18] For results obtained with the other income measures, see Appendix E, Tables E-2, E-3, and E-4.

TABLE 9
Demand Curves for All Whites in the Labor Force
($N = 1,770$)

Dependent Variable	ln $Y4$	ln W	E	i	Sex	ln FS	$\bar{R}^2$
ln H^a	.019	.060	.022	−.007	−.041	−.032	.106
	(.84)	(2.96)	(6.76)	(−8.58)	(−1.58)	(−1.37)	
−ln $WLD1$	−.092	.277	.066	−.009	.150	.216	.008
	(−.52)	(1.75)	(2.65)	(−1.18)	(.75)	(1.20)	
−ln RAD	−.294	.144	.060	−.006	−.156	.348	.005
	(−1.56)	(.85)	(2.15)	(−.87)	(−.75)	(1.87)	
ln M	.521	.014	.025	.012	.507	−.280	.043
	(4.66)	(.14)	(1.53)	(3.03)	(4.01)	(−2.48)	

[a] The health stock series is 1 = poor, 2 = fair, 3 = good, 6 = excellent. It is based on average medical outlays of all whites in each of the four health status categories.

dependent variables in the flow demand curves are $-WLD1$ and $-RAD$. All regression coefficients have been converted into elasticities or percentage changes by multiplying by $1/\overline{WLD1}$ or by $1/\overline{RAD1}$. These elasticities or percentage changes, and not the actual regression coefficients, appear in the table.[19]

When the model is estimated for the entire white labor force, the $\bar{R}^2$ in the flow demand curves fall dramatically. In Table 2, the work-loss days regression that employs $Y4$ as the income measure has an $\bar{R}^2$ of .080, and the restricted-activity days regression has an $\bar{R}^2$ of .058. In Table 9, these $\bar{R}^2$ equal .008 and .005, respectively.[20] Despite the differences in explanatory power, the regression coefficients of the four main independent variables—age, education, the wage rate, and family income—are generally consistent with those previously obtained. The two sets of coefficients tend to have the same signs and magnitudes and also tend to be statistically significant at similar levels of confidence. There are,

[19] When many of the observations on a dependent variable equal zero, probit analysis should, in principle, be applied. This technique was not employed because it was felt the costs would greatly outweigh the benefits. For a description of probit analysis, see James Tobin, "Estimation of Relationships for Limited Dependent Variables," *Econometrica*, 26, No. 1 (January 1958).

[20] Strictly speaking, the $\bar{R}^2$ in the two tables are not comparable because different forms of the dependent variable are utilized. When the arithmetic value of sick time replaces the natural logarithm as the dependent variable in the regression in Table 2, the $\bar{R}^2$ falls slightly. It is still, however, much larger than the one in Table 9.

TABLE 10

Demand Curves for Males with Positive Sick Time

(N = 406)

Dependent Variable	ln $Y4$	ln W	E	i	ln FS	$\bar{R}^2$
ln H[a]	.041	.111	.028	−.010	.018	.193
	(.76)	(2.13)	(4.01)	(−5.89)	(.41)	
−ln $WLD1$	−.040	.434	.052	−.012	.314	.118
	(−.27)	(3.06)	(2.77)	(−2.69)	(2.63)	
−ln RAD	−.138	.339	.047	−.014	.257	.082
	(−.91)	(2.32)	(2.40)	(−3.06)	(2.09)	
ln M	.869	−.369	.027	.025	−.314	.082
	(3.92)	(−1.73)	(.94)	(3.76)	(−1.75)	

[a] The health stock series is 1 = poor, 1.6 = fair, 2.9 = good, 4.9 = excellent. It is based on average medical outlays of males in each of the four health status categories.

however, three exceptions. The wage elasticity of medical care is positive in Table 9, the wage elasticity of −RAD is not significant at conventional levels, and the age coefficients in the flow demand curves are not significant.

Since persons with no sick time have similar characteristics compared to those with positive sick time—the same mean level of education, the same average wage, etc.—the model cannot explain the behavior of the former group. Even though the model cannot explain their behavior, the relationships computed when this group was excluded from the analysis are not destroyed when they are included. This finding should strengthen our confidence in the conclusions reached in Section 1.

Males

Table 10 shows demand curves for white males with positive sick time. The income variable in these demand functions is $Y4$.[21] Demand curves were also fitted for females, but the results were generally unsatisfactory and are not included in the text.[22] The regressions reveal that the effects of the exogenous variables on the demand for health and medical care are not altered by restricting the sample to males. Two points are worth noting about the magnitudes of these effects. First, the negative

[21] Results obtained with the other income measures appear in Appendix E, Tables E-5, E-6, and E-7.

[22] For the female demand curves, see Appendix E, Tables E-8, E-9, and E-10.

relation between age and health and the positive relation between age and medical care are strengthened when females are excluded. Second, the male wage elasticities of health are larger than the elasticities for males and females combined.

A tentative explanation of the first result is that the percentage rate of increase in the rate of depreciation over the life cycle is larger for men than for women. A tentative explanation of the second is that with education held constant, the correlation between the wage rate and nonmarket ability rises when females are removed from the sample. Since women are typically secondary members of the labor force, their wage might be less closely correlated with their nonmarket ability. In addition, it might not adequately reflect the monetary value they attach to an increase in their total time.

JOINT PRODUCTION AND
THE MORTALITY DATA

The empirical results in Chapter V suggest that the income elasticity of healthy days is negative. In this chapter, I offer a theoretical explanation of the negative income effect and assess whether it is present when ill health is measured by the mortality rate. In the first section, I trace the apparent inferiority of health to the existence of "joint production" in the nonmarket sector of the economy. I show that even if the "pure" income effect is positive, as the consumption model predicts, or zero, as the investment model predicts, the observed correlation between health and income might be negative. Using states of the United States as the basic units of observation, the second section offers a direct test of the joint production hypothesis. It also quantifies the relationships between the mortality rate and the principal independent variables utilized in Chapter V. Compared to health status, work-loss days, or restricted-activity days, the mortality rate is a rather extreme indicator of ill health. The death rate is, however, a more objective index than the other three. Consequently, the empirical results obtained with it are presented primarily as a *check* against those obtained with the other measures.

1. THE THEORY OF JOINT PRODUCTION

The formulation of the investment and consumption models assumed that medical care and own time were the only inputs in the gross investment production function. In reality, this function contains a vector of additional market goods that affects the quantity of gross investment produced. The variables in this vector include diet, exercise, recreation, housing, cigarettes, liquor, and rich food. Presumably, the last three goods have *negative* marginal products in the investment production function. These goods are purchased by consumers because they are also inputs into the production of other commodities, such as "smoking pleasure," that yield positive utility. Similarly, beneficial inputs like housing services produce both health and shelter Since a given input can enter more than one production function, joint production occurs in the household.

To incorporate joint production into the analysis, let the set of household production functions be[1]

$$I = I(M, X_1, X_2)$$

$$Z_1 = Z_1(X_1)$$

$$Z_2 = Z_2(X_2) \tag{6-1}$$

$$Z_j = Z_j(X_j) \qquad j = 3, \ldots, m$$

The input X_1 is a market good that increases gross investment, and the input X_2 is a good that reduces it.[2] Hence, $\partial I / \partial X_1 > 0$ and $\partial I / \partial X_2 < 0$. Note that the type of joint production considered here arises only if X_1 or X_2 *cannot* be divided into two components, one used entirely to produce Z_1 or Z_2 and the other used together with M to produce I.[3] Note also that instead of putting X_1 and X_2 in the gross investment function, one could let them affect the rate of depreciation on the stock of health. This approach has not been taken because a general model of joint production, one that is applicable to durable and nondurable household commodities, is desired.

Even though X_1 and X_2 are inputs in the gross investment production function, the marginal or average cost of gross investment does not directly depend on these two goods or their prices. This follows because when the utility function is maximized with respect to health capital or gross investment, Z_1 and Z_2 (and hence X_1 and X_2) must be held constant.[4] It is true, however, that, with M constant, an increase in X_1 or X_2 will

[1] Equation (6-1) decomposes the aggregate commodity Z into m individual commodities. For simplicity, time inputs and the stock of human capital are omitted from the production functions. The general conclusions reached in this section would not be altered if these variables were included in the analysis.

[2] In other words, market goods that improve health are aggregated into a composite input, X_1, and goods that damage health are aggregated into another composite input, X_2.

[3] Mathematically, the joint production problem discussed in the text does not arise if

$$I = I(M, X_{11}, X_{21})$$

$$Z_1 = Z_1(X_{12})$$

$$Z_2 = Z_2(X_{22}),$$

where $X_1 = X_{11} + X_{12}$ and $X_2 = X_{21} + X_{22}$.

[4] The above principle is valid even if health does not enter the utility function. Since health influences the full wealth budget constraint, a Lagrangian function must be partially differentiated with respect to H, Z_1, and Z_2. See Appendix A, equation (A-1), for this Lagrangian function.

alter the marginal product of medical care and the marginal cost of gross investment.

The relationship between X_1 or X_2 and marginal cost is now examined, and it is shown how these relationships can generate a correlation between income and marginal cost. Instead of developing the theory of joint production in detail, a specific production function is utilized:[5]

$$\ln I = \ln M + \alpha'(\ln X_1 - \ln X_2), \tag{6-2}$$

where α' is the elasticity of gross investment with respect to X_1. This production function is homogenous of degree one in medical care[6] and in all three inputs taken together. It also implies that the absolute value of the negative elasticity of I with respect to X_2 equals the elasticity of I with respect to X_1. Equation (6-2) is consistent with a common assumption in economics: If all relevant inputs are considered, then a production function will exhibit constant returns to scale.

From equation (6-2), the natural logarithm of the marginal product of medical care is

$$\ln \frac{\partial I}{\partial M} = \alpha'(\ln X_1 - \ln X_2), \tag{6-3}$$

and the natural logarithm of the marginal cost of gross investment is

$$\ln \pi = \ln P - \ln \frac{\partial I}{\partial M} = \ln P + \alpha'(\ln X_2 - \ln X_1). \tag{6-4}$$

These equations suggest that with M and Z_2 constant, an increase in X_1 will increase the marginal product of medical care and reduce the marginal cost of gross investment. On the other hand, an increase in X_2 will reduce the marginal product of medical care and increase the marginal cost of gross investment. Hence, in the terminology of the literature on production functions, X_1 and M are complements, while X_2 and M are substitutes. The equations also show that the marginal product of medical care and the marginal cost of gross investment depend only on the ratio of X_2 to X_1. In particular, this ratio is negatively correlated with the former variable and positively correlated with the latter.

[5] For a general development of the model, see Michael Grossman, "The Economics of Joint Production in the Household," University of Chicago, Center for Mathematical Studies in Business and Economics, mimeographed, 1971.

[6] If M were viewed as a composite input representing both medical care and own time, equation (6-2) would be consistent with diminishing marginal productivity of medical care.

Suppose income increases, with the prices of market goods and own time, the interest rate, the rate of depreciation on the stock of health, and the efficiency of nonmarket production all held fixed. Under these conditions, will the shadow price of health remain constant? To answer this question, differentiate equation (6-4) with respect to the natural logarithm of income:

$$\eta_\pi = \alpha'(\eta_2 - \eta_1). \tag{6-5}$$

In this equation, η_π is the income elasticity of marginal cost, η_2 is the income elasticity of X_2 or Z_2, and η_1 is the income elasticity of X_1 or Z_1. The equation reveals that marginal cost is independent of income only if Z_1 and Z_2 have the same income elasticities. In general, $\eta_\pi \gtreqless 0$ as $\eta_2 \gtreqless \eta_1$. This follows because the correlation between X_2/X_1 and income depends on the magnitude of η_2 compared to η_1. Given $\eta_2 > \eta_1$, this ratio would rise with income, which would lower the marginal product of medical care and raise marginal cost. The reverse would occur if $\eta_1 > \eta_2$.

Provided $\eta_1 \neq \eta_2$, health would have a nonzero income elasticity even if it were solely an investment commodity. That is, an increase in income would change the marginal cost of gross investment, shift the MEC schedule, and alter the demand for health. In the investment model, the income elasticity of health would be given by[7]

$$\eta_H = \varepsilon\alpha'(\eta_1 - \eta_2), \tag{6-6}$$

and it is clear that $\eta_H < 0$ if $\eta_2 > \eta_1$.[8] Thus, the observed negative income elasticity of healthy days can be explained without resorting to the argument that health is an inferior commodity. Instead, one interpretation of this finding is that the detrimental inputs in the gross investment production function have higher income elasticities than the beneficial inputs. In fact, existing consumer budget studies indicate that alcohol consumption is very income elastic ($\eta = 1.6$), although cigarette smoking is not ($\eta = .6$).[9] The income elasticity of total food consumption

[7] Since $\ln(r + \delta) = \ln W + \ln G - \ln \pi$, $\eta_H = \varepsilon\eta_\pi$. Substitution of equation (6-5) for η_π yields equation (6-6).

[8] In the pure consumption model, health might have a negative income elasticity if $\eta_2 > \eta_1$, but this is not a sufficient condition. Instead, the substitution effect introduced by joint production would have to outweigh the positive income effect that would be observed in its absence. For an elaboration of this argument, see Grossman, "The Economics of Joint Production."

[9] For one set of estimates of income elasticities for items that exhaust total consumption, see Robert T. Michael, *The Effect of Education on Efficiency in Consumption*, New York, NBER, Occasional Paper 116, 1972.

is fairly small ($\eta = .6$), but rich and caloric varieties of food might have large elasticities. In addition, other market goods that as yet have not been identified might have large income elasticities and harmful effects on health.

If the consumption of X_2 were more responsive to changes in income than the consumption of X_1, health would be negatively correlated with income in the investment model. This does not mean that medical care would also have a negative income elasticity. In particular, wealthier persons might have an incentive to offset *part* of the reduction in health caused by an increase in X_2/X_1 by increasing their medical outlays. One easily shows that the income elasticity of medical care would equal[10]

$$\eta_M = \alpha'(\eta_1 - \eta_2)(\varepsilon - 1). \tag{6-7}$$

Assume $\eta_2 > \eta_1$ so that η_H is negative. Then according to equation (6-7), η_M would be positive if the elasticity of the MEC schedule were less than unity. Given this condition, wealthier persons would simultaneously reduce their demand for health but increase their demand for medical care. These are precisely the relationships that were observed in Chapter V.

One final comment on the effects of joint production is in order. The law of the downward sloping demand curve, the most fundamental law in economics, indicates that the quantity of X_2 demanded would be negatively correlated with its price. So an increase in $P2$, the price of X_2, would raise the marginal product of medical care, lower the marginal cost of gross investment, and increase the demand for health. A formula for the elasticity of health with respect to $P2$ is

$$e_{P2} = -\varepsilon\alpha'e_2, \tag{6-8}$$

where e_2 is the price elasticity of demand for X_2 (defined to be positive).[11] Since e_{P2} exceeds zero, health and X_2 are substitutes. On the other hand, an increase in $P1$, the price of X_1, would lower the marginal product of medical care, raise marginal cost, and reduce the demand for health. Consequently, health and X_1 are complements. This formulation suggests a direct test of the joint production hypothesis. If $P1$ and $P2$ entered the

[10] Since $\ln M = \ln I + \alpha'(\ln X_2 - \ln X_1)$ and since $\eta_I = \eta_H$, $\eta_M = \eta_H + \alpha'(\eta_2 - \eta_1)$. Substitution of equation (6-6) for η_H yields equation (6-7).

[11] From the definition of the monetary rate of return on an investment in health, $e_{P2} = -\varepsilon(d \ln \pi/d \ln P2)$. Differentiating equation (6-4) with respect to $\ln P2$, one gets $d \ln \pi/d \ln P2 = -\alpha'e_2$. Substituting the last equation into the expression for e_{P2}, one has equation (6-8). This derivation assumes that the demand for X_1 is independent of the price of X_2.

set of exogenous variables in the health demand curve, then the regression coefficient of $P1$ should be negative, and the coefficient of $P2$ should be positive.

2. THE MORTALITY DATA

This section presents estimates of health demand functions in which ill health is measured by the mortality rate. The basic units of observation are 48 of the 50 states of the United States (Alaska and Hawaii are excluded) for the year 1960. The transition from individual data to data grouped by states is made by postulating homoscedasticity at the individual level. This implies that each observation should be weighted by the square root of the state's population.[12]

The specific mortality variable employed is the crude death rate of the white population, d. This variable essentially measures the fraction of the people in a given state who had no healthy days or 365 sick days in 1960.[13] Since d is analogous to TL and since the investment model suggests $-\ln TL$ should be the dependent variable in the health flow demand curve, the dependent variable in the mortality regressions is $-\ln d$. To take account of variations in the crude death rate due to variations in age and sex population distributions across states, an expected death rate, $\bar{d}$, enters the regressions as one of the independent variables. This variable was computed by applying U.S. age-sex specific death rates of whites to age-sex population distributions of whites in each state. It is described in more detail in Appendix F.

The other exogenous variables include family income, the wage rate, education, average hourly earnings of paramedical personnel (all members of the health industry excluding doctors) adjusted for quality (PN), and the price of cigarettes per pack (PC).[14] Hourly earnings of paramedical personnel are employed as an index of the price of medical care. In principle, this index should also take account of variations in the price of physicians' services across states. Unfortunately, data on physicians'

[12] See E. Malinvaud, *Statistical Methods of Econometrics*, Amsterdam, 1966, pp. 242–246. The coefficients obtained from unweighted regressions (not shown) are fairly similar to the weighted regression coefficients presented in this section.

[13] This assumes that all deaths occurred at the beginning of the year. If this were not the case, the above interpretation of d would still be valid provided a long period of illness preceded death.

[14] The regressions in the text exclude family size from the set of exogenous variables. When it was included, its own regression coefficient was extremely small, and the other coefficients were not affected.

income for the year 1960 are not readily available. The price of cigarettes measures the price of one of the detrimental inputs in the gross investment production function. The prices of other inputs in the production function are assumed to be constant. This assumption is advanced because these inputs are difficult to identify and because information on their prices is virtually nonexistent.[15] Detailed definitions of all the exogenous variables and the data sources from which they were taken are discussed in Appendix F.

Table 11 shows the mortality demand curves. Since family income and the wage rate are very highly correlated ($r = .946$), the table contains three regressions. The first one includes both these variables, the second omits the wage, and the third omits income. The $\bar{R}^2$ are large in all three regressions because the expected death rate is one of the independent variables. Preliminary regressions with $-\ln(d/\bar{d})$ as the dependent variable yielded $\bar{R}^2$ equal to .6.[16] The regression coefficients and t ratios of the other independent variables were almost identical, however, to those in Table 11.

TABLE 11
Demand for Health in States of the United States, 1960

Regression Number	ln Y	ln W	E	$-\ln \bar{d}$	ln PN	ln PC	$\bar{R}^2$
1	−.496	.332	.054	.842	−.330	.019	.913
	(−4.48)	(2.83)	(6.51)	(15.32)	(−2.71)	(.25)	
2	−.226		.056	.916	−.252	−.008	.898
	(−3.71)		(6.25)	(15.45)	(−1.96)	(−.10)	
3		−.120	.057	.867	−.422	−.038	.873
		(−1.66)	(5.68)	(13.55)	(−2.92)	(−.43)	

NOTE: In all regressions, the dependent variable is $-\ln d$.

Regression 1 reveals that income, the wage, and education have the *same effects* on mortality as they do on sick time. Income is positively correlated with these two measures of ill health, the wage is negatively

[15] I computed an implicit price of liquor by dividing expenditures by a quantity index (total absolute alcohol content in gallons of sales per person of drinking age). When the quantity index was regressed on income and price, the estimated price elasticity was zero. For this reason, the price variable was excluded from the mortality regressions.

[16] This form assumes that the elasticity of d with respect to $\bar{d}$ equals one.

correlated with them, and so is education.[17] Moreover, the magnitudes of the coefficients in regression 1 are fairly similar to the magnitudes of the corresponding coefficients in the NORC health flow demand curves. For example, if all other variables were held constant, a one-year increase in the level of formal schooling would reduce the white mortality and sick time rates by approximately 5.4 and 4.6 percent. To cite another illustration, the wage elasticities of $-d$, $-WLD1$, and $-RAD$ equal .332, .471, and .341, respectively.[18]

Not all the empirical results of the mortality analysis are in complete agreement with those of the NORC analysis. The negative income elasticity of $-d$ is approximately twice as large as the income elasticity of sick time ($-.496$ compared with $-.177$ when $-TL = -WLD1$ or $-.226$ when $-TL = -RAD$). Hence, although the NORC wage elasticity of health is larger than the absolute value of the income elasticity, the reverse is true in the mortality demand curve. In addition, regressions 2 and 3 show that if either income or the wage is excluded from the set of independent variables, the remaining variable has a negative elasticity. On the other hand, the gross wage and income elasticities of health are positive in the NORC sample.

In one sense, the finding that the death rate is positively related to income and negatively related to the wage rate is due to the extremely high correlation between ln Y and ln W ($r = .946$). When a dependent variable is regressed on two such highly correlated variables, it can be easily proven that their regression coefficients are bound to have opposite signs.[19] In another sense, however, this finding is important from a theoretical point of view. Suppose one did not have a theory to explain

[17] Using the same basic data, Victor R. Fuchs and Richard D. Auster, Irving Leveson, and Deborah Sarachek found a positive correlation between income and mortality and a negative correlation between education and mortality. See Fuchs, "Some Economic Aspects of Mortality in the United States," New York, NBER, mimeographed, 1965; and Auster, Leveson, and Sarachek, "The Production of Health, an Exploratory Study," *Journal of Human Resources*, 4, No. 4 (Fall 1969), and reprinted as Chapter 8 in Victor R. Fuchs (ed.), *Essays in the Economics of Health and Medical Care*, New York, NBER, 1972. The main difference between my analysis and that of Fuchs and Auster, Leveson, and Sarachek is that I emphasize the demand curve for health, while they emphasize the production function.

[18] The wage elasticities of $-WLD1$ and $-RAD$, as well as the income elasticities cited in the next paragraph, are taken from Table 6.

[19] See Reuben Gronau, "The Effect of Traveling Time on the Demand for Passenger Airline Transportation," unpublished Ph.D. dissertation, Columbia University, Chapter 6. In general, if the two variables in question have positive simple correlation coefficients with the dependent variable, then the one with the larger correlation would exhibit a positive coefficient in the multiple regression.

the forces influencing the demand for health. Then he could not predict whether income or the wage would be more likely to have a negative effect on mortality. Since the value of the marginal product of health capital is more closely related to the wage than to income, the investment model would predict a negative wage elasticity of the death rate. This is precisely what is observed empirically.[20]

The first regression in Table 11 indicates that the two price variables have the "correct signs" in the mortality demand curve. An increase in the price of paramedical personnel, which represents an increase in the marginal cost of gross investment, reduces the quantity of health demanded. The computed elasticity of $-d$ with respect to PN is $-.330$. In accordance with the notion that the shadow price of health is negatively correlated with the price of cigarettes, this price has a positive health elasticity. This elasticity is small ($e_{P2} = .019$), and unfortunately, it is not statistically significant. Moreover, it becomes negative when either income or the wage is excluded from the regressions. Since $e_{P2} = \varepsilon\alpha'e_2$ and since $\varepsilon = .5$, e_{P2} would be small if the demand for cigarettes were price-inelastic.[21] Based on the state data, e_2 equals .4, which implies that α' equals .1. That is, a 1 percent increase in cigarette smoking would reduce the marginal product of medical care by one-tenth of 1 percent. This estimate of α' coincides with a direct calculation of the elasticity of the mortality rate with respect to cigarette consumption made by Auster, Leveson, and Sarachek.[22]

In summary, the remarkable qualitative and quantitative agreement between the mortality and sick time regression results should strengthen our confidence in the health measures utilized in Chapter V and in the way these measures have been interpreted. Even though the mortality rate is a more objective measure of ill health than sick time, variations in income, education, and the wage rate have similar effects on these two indexes. Perhaps the most striking finding in this study is that health has a negative income elasticity. One explanation of this result is that the income elasticities of the detrimental inputs in the health production

[20] Morris Silver should again be credited with stressing the importance of the wage variable in the health demand curve. He argues that health is a time-intensive *consumption* commodity and that an increase in W should increase the death rate. See "An Econometric Analysis of Spatial Variations in Mortality by Race and Sex," in Fuchs (ed.), *op. cit.*, Chap. 9.

[21] In addition, the health elasticity of the price of cigarettes might be small because knowledge about the detrimental effects of smoking was not widespread prior to the issuance of the Surgeon General's report on health and smoking in 1964.

[22] See "The Production of Health," Tables 3 and 4.

function exceed those of the beneficial inputs, although the evidence in support of this view is by no means overwhelming. Future research should attempt to identify the harmful inputs and assess how sensitive their consumption is to changes in the level of income.

3. GLOSSARY

X_1 A market good with a positive marginal product in the gross investment production function

X_2 A market good with a negative marginal product in the gross investment production function

α' Elasticity of gross investment with respect to X_1

$-\alpha'$ Elasticity of gross investment with respect to X_2

η_π Income elasticity of marginal cost

η_1 Income elasticity of X_1

η_2 Income elasticity of X_2

η_H Income elasticity of health

η_M Income elasticity of medical care

$P1$ Price of X_1

$P2$ Price of X_2

e_2 Price elasticity of X_2

e_{P2} Health elasticity of P_2

d Crude death rate, states of the United States

$\bar{d}$ Expected death rate

PN Price of paramedical personnel

PC Price of cigarettes

Appendix A

UTILITY MAXIMIZATIONS

1. DISCRETE TIME

To maximize utility subject to the full wealth and production function constraints, form the Lagrangian expression

$$L = U(\phi_0 H_0, \ldots, \phi_n H_n, Z_0, \ldots, Z_n) + \lambda \left[R - \sum \frac{C_i + C_{1i} + W_i TL_i}{(1 + r)^i} \right],$$

(A-1)

where $C_i = P_i M_i + W_i TH_i$ and $C_{1i} = F_i X_i + W_i T_i$. Differentiating L with respect to gross investment in period $i - 1$ and setting the partial derivative equal to zero, one obtains

$$Uh_i \frac{\partial h_i}{\partial H_i} \frac{\partial H_i}{\partial I_{i-1}} + Uh_{i+1} \frac{\partial h_{i+1}}{\partial H_{i+1}} \frac{\partial H_{i+1}}{\partial I_{i-1}} + \ldots + Uh_n \frac{\partial h_n}{\partial H_n} \frac{\partial H_n}{\partial I_{i-1}}$$

$$= \lambda \left[\frac{(dC_{i-1}/dI_{i-1})}{(1 + r)^{i-1}} + \frac{W_i(\partial TL_i/\partial H_i)(\partial H_i/\partial I_{i-1})}{(1 + r)^i} \right.$$

$$+ \frac{W_{i+1}(\partial TL_{i+1}/\partial H_{i+1})(\partial H_{i+1}/\partial I_{i-1})}{(1 + r)^{i+1}} + \ldots$$

$$\left. + \frac{W_n(\partial TL_n/\partial H_n)(\partial H_n/\partial I_{i-1})}{(1 + r)^n} \right].$$

(A-2)

But $\partial h_i/\partial H_i = G_i$, $\partial H_i/\partial I_{i-1} = 1$, $\partial H_{i+1}/\partial I_{i-1} = (1 - \delta_i)$, $\partial H_n/\partial I_{i-1} = (1 - \delta_i) \ldots (1 - \delta_{n-1})$, $dC_{i-1}/dI_{i-1} = \pi_{i-1}$, and $\partial TL_i/\partial H_i = -G_i$. Therefore,

$$\frac{\pi_{i-1}}{(1 + r)^{i-1}} = \frac{W_i G_i}{(1 + r)^i} + \frac{(1 - \delta_i)W_{i+1}G_{i+1}}{(1 + r)^{i+1}} + \ldots$$

$$+ \frac{(1 - \delta_i) \ldots (1 - \delta_{n-1})W_n G_n}{(1 + r)^n} + \frac{Uh_i}{\lambda} G_i$$

$$+ (1 - \delta_i)\frac{Uh_{i+1}}{\lambda}G_{i+1} + \dots$$

$$+ (1 - \delta_i) \dots (1 - \delta_{n-1})\frac{Uh_n}{\lambda}G_n. \tag{A-3}$$

2. CONTINUOUS TIME

Let the utility function be

$$U = \int m_i f(\phi_i H_i, Z_i)\,di, \tag{A-4}$$

where m_i is the weight attached to utility in period i. Equation (A-4) defines an additive utility function, but any monotonic transformation of this function could be employed.[1] Let all household production functions be homogeneous of degree one. Then $C_i = \pi_i I_i$, $C_{1i} = q_i Z_i$, and full wealth can be written as

$$R = \int e^{-ri}(\pi_i I_i + q_i Z_i + W_i T L_i)\,di. \tag{A-5}$$

By definition,

$$I_i = \dot{H}_i + \delta_i H_i, \tag{A-6}$$

where $\dot{H}_i$ is the instantaneous rate of change of capital stock. Substitution of (A-6) into (A-5) yields

$$R = \int e^{ri}(\pi_i \delta_i H_i + \pi_i \dot{H}_i + q_i Z_i + W_i T L_i)\,di. \tag{A-7}$$

To maximize the utility function, form the Lagrangian

$$L - \lambda R = \int [m_i f(\phi_i H_i, Z_i) - \lambda e^{-ri}(\pi_i \delta_i H_i + \pi_i \dot{H}_i + q_i Z_i + W_i T L_i)]\,di, \tag{A-8}$$

or

$$L - \lambda R = \int J(H_i, \dot{H}_i, Z_i, i)\,di, \tag{A-9}$$

[1] Robert H. Strotz has shown, however, that certain restrictions must be placed on the m_i. In particular, the initial consumption plan will be fulfilled if and only if $m_i = (m_0)^i$. See "Myopia and Inconsistency in Dynamic Utility Maximization," *Review of Economic Studies*, 23, No. 62 (1955–56).

where

$$J = m_i f(\phi_i H_i, Z_i) - \lambda\, e^{-ri}(\pi_i \delta_i H_i + \pi_i \dot{H}_i + q_i Z_i + W_i T L_i). \quad \text{(A-10)}$$

Euler's equation for the optimal path of H_i is

$$\frac{\partial J}{\partial H_i} = \frac{d}{di} \frac{\partial J}{\partial \dot{H}_i} \qquad \text{(A-11)}$$

In the present context,

$$\frac{\partial J}{\partial H_i} = U h_i G_i - \lambda\, e^{-ri} \pi_i \delta_i + \lambda\, e^{-ri} W_i G_i,$$

$$\frac{\partial J}{\partial \dot{H}_i} = -\lambda\, e^{-ri} \pi_i,$$

and

$$\frac{d}{di} \frac{\partial J}{\partial \dot{H}_i} = -\lambda\, e^{-ri} \dot{\pi}_i + \lambda\, e^{-ri} r \pi_i. \qquad \text{(A-12)}$$

Consequently,

$$G_i[W_i + (U h_i/\lambda)\, e^{ri}] = \pi_i(r - \tilde{\pi}_i + \delta_i), \qquad \text{(A-13)}$$

which is the continuous time analogue of equation (1-13).

Appendix B

DERIVATION OF INVESTMENT MODEL FORMULAS

1. THE INVESTMENT DEMAND CURVE

To find the optimal amount of I_{i-1} in the pure investment model, redefine the full wealth constraint as

$$R' = A_0 + \sum \frac{W_i h_i - \pi_i I_i}{(1 + r)^i}. \tag{B-1}$$

Maximization of R' with respect to I_{i-1} yields

$$\frac{\partial R'}{\partial I_{i-1}} - 0 = \frac{W_i G_i}{(1 + r)^i} + \frac{(1 - \delta_i) W_{i+1} G_{i+1}}{(1 + r)^{i+1}} + \ldots$$
$$+ \frac{(1 - \delta_i) \ldots (1 - \delta_{n-1}) W_n G_n}{(1 + r)^n} - \frac{\pi_{i-1}}{(1 + r)^{i-1}}. \tag{B-2}$$

If (B-2) is combined with the first order condition for I_i by means of the technique outlined in Chapter I, Section 2, then

$$\gamma_i = \frac{W_i G_i}{\pi_{i-1}} = r - \tilde{\pi}_{i-1} + \delta_i. \tag{B-3}$$

To satisfy second order optimality conditions, it is necessary that

$$\frac{\partial^2 R'}{\partial I_{i-1}^2} < 0 = \frac{W_i(\partial G_i/\partial H_i)}{(1 + r)^i} + \frac{(1 - \delta_i)^2 W_{i+1}(\partial G_{i+1}/\partial H_{i+1})}{(1 + r)^{i+1}}$$
$$+ \ldots + \frac{[(1 - \delta_i) \ldots (1 - \delta_{n-1})]^2 W_n(\partial G_n/\partial H_n)}{(1 + r)^n},$$

or $\partial G_i/\partial H_i < 0$, all i. Diminishing marginal productivity in all periods is required because (B-3) implies that optimal H must satisfy

$$\frac{\partial \gamma_i}{\partial H_i} = \frac{W_i(\partial G_i/\partial H_i)}{\pi_{i-1}} < 0.$$

In the continuous time model, R' is given by

$$R' = \int e^{-ri}(W_i h_i - \pi_i I_i)\, di, \tag{B-4}$$

or

$$R' = \int e^{-ri}(W_i h_i - \pi_i \delta_i H_i - \pi_i \dot{H}_i)\, di. \tag{B-5}$$

Hence,

$$R' = \int J(H_i, \dot{H}_i, i)\, di, \tag{B-6}$$

where $J = e^{-ri}(W_i h_i - \pi_i \delta_i H_i - \pi_i \dot{H}_i)$. Using the Euler equation outlined in Appendix A, one derives the condition for the optimal path of health capital over the life cycle:

$$\gamma_i = \frac{W_i G_i}{\pi_i} = r - \tilde{\pi}_i + \delta_i. \tag{B-7}$$

In Chapter II, it was indicated that certain production functions of healthy time might exhibit increasing or constant marginal productivity in some regions (see footnote 2). Suppose, for example, that healthy time increased at an increasing rate in the vicinity of the death stock, as in Figure B-1. Then quantities of $H < H^*$ would never be observed because the MEC schedule would be upward sloping in the range $H_{min} < H_i < H^*$.

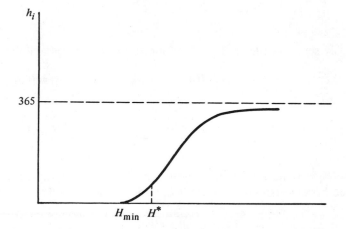

Figure B-1

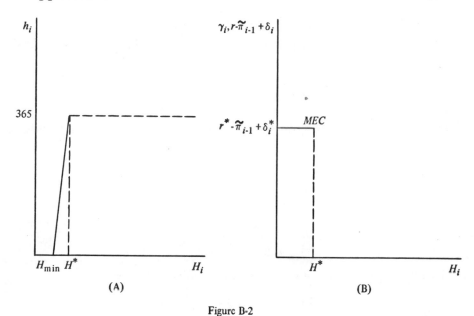

Figure B-2

This implies that individuals would choose an infinite life. Since observed behavior is consistent with finite life spans, segments of increasing marginal productivity can be ruled out around the death age.[1]

Production functions with constant marginal productivity are somewhat more difficult to discard. In panel A of Figure B-2, the number of healthy days is proportional to the stock of health until $H_i = H^*$. Since G_i is constant for $H_i < H^*$ and zero thereafter, the MEC schedule has a discontinuity when $H_i = H^*$. If the cost of health capital were less than $r^* - \tilde{\pi}^*_{i-1} + \delta^*_i$ in panel B, H^* would be the equilibrium stock of health and 365 days would be the equilibrium number of healthy days. At $r - \tilde{\pi}_{i-1} + \delta_i = r^* - \tilde{\pi}^*_{i-1} + \delta^*_i$, any stock between H_{min} and H^* would be optimal, while a higher cost of capital would give rise to an equilibrium stock H_{min}. Although the production function in panel A is not inconsistent with observed behavior, it may be ruled out because "nature does not make jumps." That is, it is reasonable to assume healthy time reaches its upper limit gradually and in a manner that rules out discontinuities in the MEC schedule.

[1] In general, if the production function had alternating segments of increasing and diminishing marginal productivity, the ones with increasing marginal productivity would never be observed.

2. VARIATIONS IN DEPRECIATION RATES

All formulas that were employed to study the effects of life cycle variations in depreciation rates were proved in Chapter II. Therefore, this section develops formulas for the analysis of variations in δ_i among individuals of the same age. If $\tilde{\pi}_{i-1} = 0$, all i, then

$$\ln (r + \delta_i) = \ln W_i + \ln G_i - \ln \pi. \tag{B-8}$$

Differentiation of (B-8) with respect to $\ln \delta_i$ yields

$$\frac{\delta_i}{r + \delta_i} = \frac{\partial \ln G_i}{\partial \ln H_i} \frac{d \ln H_i}{d \ln \delta_i},$$

or

$$\frac{d \ln H_i}{d \ln \delta_i} = -s_i \varepsilon. \tag{B-9}$$

The natural logarithm of gross investment may be written

$$\ln I_i = \ln H_i + \ln (\tilde{H}_i + \delta_i). \tag{B-10}$$

Hence,

$$\frac{d \ln I_i}{d \ln \delta_i} = \frac{d \ln H_i}{d \ln \delta_i} + \frac{\delta_i + (d\tilde{H}_i/d \ln \delta_i)}{\tilde{H}_i + \delta_i}.$$

It was shown in Chapter II that $\tilde{H}_i = -s_i \varepsilon \tilde{\delta}$. Thus, $d\tilde{H}_i/d \ln \delta_i = -s_i(1 - s_i)\varepsilon \tilde{\delta}$. Utilizing (B-9) and the last two expressions, one has

$$\frac{d \ln I_i}{d \ln \delta_i} = \frac{(1 - s_i \varepsilon)(\delta_i - s_i \varepsilon \tilde{\delta}) + s_i^2 \varepsilon \tilde{\delta}}{\delta_i - s_i \varepsilon \tilde{\delta}}. \tag{B-11}$$

3. MARKET AND NONMARKET EFFICIENCY

Wage Effects

To obtain the wage elasticities of medical care and the time spent producing health, three equations must be partially differentiated with respect to the wage. These equations are the gross investment production and the two first order conditions for cost minimization:

$$I(M, TH; E) = Mg(t; E) = (\tilde{H} + \delta)H$$

$$W = \pi g'$$

$$P = \pi(g - tg').$$

Since I is linear homogeneous in M and TH,

$$\frac{\partial(g - tg')}{\partial M} = -t\frac{\partial(g - tg')}{\partial TH}$$

$$\frac{\partial g'}{\partial TH} = \frac{1}{t}\frac{\partial(g - tg')}{\partial TH}$$

$$\sigma_p = \frac{(g - tg')g'}{I\partial(g - tg')/\partial TH}.$$

Therefore, the following relationships hold:

$$\frac{\partial(g - tg')}{\partial M} = -\frac{t(g - tg')g'}{I\sigma_p}$$

$$\frac{\partial g'}{\partial TH} = -\frac{1}{t}\frac{(g - tg')g'}{I\sigma_p} \tag{B-12}$$

$$\frac{\partial(g - tg')}{\partial TH} = \frac{(g - tg')g'}{I\sigma_p}.$$

Carrying out the differentiation, one gets

$$g'\frac{dTH}{dW} + (g - tg')\frac{dM}{dW} = -\frac{H(\tilde{H} + \delta)\varepsilon}{\pi}\left(\frac{d\pi}{dW} - \frac{\pi}{W}\right)$$

$$1 = g'\frac{d\pi}{dW} + \pi\left(\frac{\partial g'}{\partial TH}\frac{dTH}{dW} + \frac{\partial g'}{\partial M}\frac{dM}{dW}\right)$$

$$0 = (g - tg')\frac{d\pi}{dW} + \pi\left[\frac{\partial(g - tg')}{\partial TH}\frac{dTH}{dW} + \frac{\partial(g - tg')}{\partial M}\frac{dM}{dW}\right].$$

Using the cost-minimization conditions and (B-12) and rearranging terms, one has

$$I\varepsilon\frac{d\pi}{dW} + W\frac{dTH}{dW} + P\frac{dM}{dW} = \frac{I\varepsilon\pi}{W}$$

$$I\sigma_p\frac{d\pi}{dW} - \frac{1}{t}P\frac{dTH}{dW} + P\frac{dM}{dW} = I\frac{\pi}{W}\sigma_p \tag{B-13}$$

$$I\sigma_p\frac{d\pi}{dW} + W\frac{dTH}{dW} - tW\frac{dM}{dW} = 0.$$

Since (B-13) is a system of three equations in three unknowns, dTH/dW, dM/dW, and $d\pi/dW$, Cramer's rule can be applied to solve for, say, dM/dW:

$$\frac{dM}{dW} = \frac{\begin{vmatrix} I\varepsilon + W & +I\varepsilon\pi/W \\ I\sigma_p - (1/t)P & +I(\pi/W)\sigma_p \\ I\sigma_p + W & -0 \end{vmatrix}}{\begin{vmatrix} I\varepsilon + W & +P \\ I\sigma_p - (1/t)P & +P \\ I\sigma_p + W & -tW \end{vmatrix}}.$$

The determinant in the denominator reduces to $I\sigma_p\pi^2 I^2/THM$. The determinant in the numerator is

$$\frac{I\sigma_p}{THM}\left(I\pi\sigma_p THM + I\pi\varepsilon\frac{P}{W}M^2\right).$$

Therefore,

$$\frac{dM}{dW} = \frac{THM}{I\pi}\left(\sigma_p + \frac{\varepsilon P}{WTH}\right)M.$$

In elasticity notation, this becomes

$$e_{M,W} = (1 - K)\varepsilon + K\sigma_p. \tag{B-14}$$

Along similar lines, one easily shows

$$e_{TH,W} = (1 - K)(\varepsilon - \sigma_p). \tag{B-15}$$

The Role of Human Capital

To convert the change in productivity due to a shift in human capital into a change in average or marginal cost, let the percentage changes in the marginal products of medical care and own time for a one unit change in human capital be given by

$$\frac{\partial(g - tg')}{\partial E}\frac{1}{g - tg'} = \frac{g\hat{g} - tg'\hat{g}'}{g - tg'}$$

$$\frac{\partial g'}{\partial E}\frac{1}{g'} = \hat{g}'.$$

If a shift in human capital were factor-neutral, the percentage changes in these two marginal products would be equal:

$$\hat{g}' = \frac{g\hat{g} - tg'\hat{g}'}{g - tg'},$$

or

$$\hat{g}' = \hat{g} = r_H. \qquad \text{(B-16)}$$

The average cost of gross investment in health is defined as

$$\bar{\pi} = (PM + WTH)I^{-1} = (P + Wt)g^{-1}.$$

Given "factor-neutrality,"

$$\frac{d\bar{\pi}}{dE}\frac{1}{\bar{\pi}} = -\hat{g} = -r_H. \qquad \text{(B-17)}$$

This coincides with the percentage change in marginal cost since

$$\pi = P(g - tg_t)^{-1},$$

and

$$\frac{d\pi}{dE}\frac{1}{\pi} = -\left(\frac{g\hat{g} - tg'\hat{g}'}{g - tg'}\right) = -\hat{g}' = -\hat{g} = -r_H. \qquad \text{(B-18)}$$

Chapter III outlined a derivation of the human capital parameter in the demand curve for medical care but did not give a rigorous proof. Taking the *total* derivative of E in the gross investment function, one computes this parameter:

$$\frac{dI}{dE}\frac{1}{I} = \frac{M(g - tg')}{I}\hat{M} + \frac{THg'}{I}\widehat{TH} + r_H.$$

Since $\hat{M} = \widehat{TH}$ and $\hat{H} = \hat{I}$, the last equation can be rewritten as

$$\hat{H} = \hat{M} + r_H\varepsilon.$$

Solving for $\hat{M}$ and noting that $\hat{H} = r_H\varepsilon$, one gets

$$\hat{M} = r_H(\varepsilon - 1). \qquad \text{(B-19)}$$

Appendix C

DERIVATION OF CONSUMPTION MODEL FORMULAS

1. LIFE CYCLE PATTERNS

Let the utility function be

$$U = (\Sigma m^i h_i^{-B})^{-1/B} J(Z_i). \tag{C-1}$$

This is a constant elasticity of substitution function in terms of healthy time. If the flow of healthy time per unit of health capital were independent of the stock, then

$$\frac{UH_i}{UH_1} = (1 + r)^{1-i} \left(\frac{r + \delta_i}{r + \delta_1}\right) = m^{i-1} \left(\frac{H_1}{H_i}\right)^{B+1}. \tag{C-2}$$

Solving (C-2) for H_i and taking natural logarithms of the resulting expression, one gets

$$\ln H_i = \ln H_1 + \sigma(i - 1) \ln m + \sigma(i - 1) \ln (1 + r)$$
$$+ \sigma[\ln (r + \delta_1) - \ln (r + \delta_i)], \tag{C-3}$$

where $\sigma = 1/(1 + B)$. The derivative of $\ln H_i$ with respect to i is

$$\tilde{H}_i = \sigma[\ln m + \ln (1 + r) - s_i \tilde{\delta}]. \tag{C-4}$$

Note also that

$$\tilde{H}_{ii} = -s_i(1 - s_i)\sigma\tilde{\delta}^2. \tag{C-5}$$

It was shown in Chapter II that

$$\tilde{I}_i = \frac{\tilde{H}_i^2 + \tilde{H}_{ii} + \delta_i(\tilde{H}_i + \tilde{\delta})}{\tilde{H}_i + \delta_i}.$$

Substituting (C-4) and (C-5) into the last equation and assuming no time preference, one gets

$$\tilde{I}_i = \frac{\tilde{\delta}(1 - s_i\sigma)(\delta_i - s_i\sigma\tilde{\delta}) + s_i^2\sigma\tilde{\delta}^2 + r^2\sigma^2 - 2rs_i\sigma^2\tilde{\delta}^2 + \delta_i\sigma r}{\tilde{H}_i + \delta_i}. \tag{C-6}$$

If $r = 0$, equation (C-6) reduces to

$$\tilde{I}_i = \frac{\tilde{\delta}(1 - \sigma)(\delta_i - \sigma\tilde{\delta}) + \sigma\tilde{\delta}^2}{\delta_i - \sigma\tilde{\delta}}.$$

Since gross investment cannot be negative, $\delta_i > \sigma\tilde{\delta}$. Therefore, given a zero rate of interest, a sufficient condition for gross investment to be positively correlated with age is $\sigma < 1$. If r exceeds zero, it becomes somewhat more difficult to evaluate the sign of $\tilde{I}_i$. Suppose this sign is evaluated when $\tilde{H}_i$ is negative. Then the condition for positive gross investment requires that $\delta_i > s_i\sigma\tilde{\delta} - r$. This condition could hold even if $\delta_i < s_i\sigma\tilde{\delta}$. But provided the rate of interest is relatively small, it is not likely to be satisfied unless $\delta_i > s_i\sigma\tilde{\delta}$. In this situation, an elasticity of substitution less than unity would make all terms in the numerator of (C-6) positive except $-2rs_i\sigma^2\tilde{\delta}^2$. Thus, it is extremely likely that $\tilde{I}_i$ would be positive.

2. MARKET AND NONMARKET EFFICIENCY

To analyze the effects of variations in the shadow price of health among individuals of the same age, let the cross-sectional demand curve be

$$H = H(R^*, Q^*) \tag{C-7}$$

where $R^* = R/Q$ and $Q^* = (r + \delta)\pi/Q$. Differentiation of (C-7) with respect to the wage rate holding R^* fixed yields

$$\frac{dH}{dW}\frac{W}{H} = \frac{\partial H}{\partial Q^*}\frac{Q^*}{H}\frac{dQ^*}{dW}\frac{W}{Q^*}$$

$$e_{H,w} = -e_H\frac{d\ln Q^*}{d\ln W}.$$

An evaluation of the elasticity of Q^* with respect to W indicates

$$\frac{d\ln Q^*}{d\ln W} = K - \frac{d\ln Q}{d\ln W}.$$

Since $\ln Q = w \ln (r + \delta)\pi + (1 - w) \ln q$,

$$\frac{d\ln Q}{d\ln W} = wK + (1 - w)\frac{WT}{qZ} = \bar{K}.$$

Therefore,

$$\eta_{Q^*,w} = K - \bar{K}$$

and

$$e_{H,W} = -e_H(K - \bar{K}).$$ (C-8)

To compute the wage elasticity of medical care, note that

$$I(M, T) = (\tilde{H} + \delta)H.$$

The wage derivative in this equation is

$$Ie_H\frac{d\pi}{dW} + W\frac{dTH}{dW} + P\frac{dM}{dW} = Ie_H\bar{K}\frac{\pi}{W}.$$

This becomes the first equation in (B-13). The second and third equations remain the same, and the solution of the system is

$$e_{M,W} = K\sigma_p - (K - \bar{K})e_H.$$ (C-9)

By differentiating the demand function (C-7) with money full wealth and the wage rate fixed, the human capital parameter in the demand curve for health is calculated:

$$\frac{dH}{dE}\frac{1}{H} = \frac{\partial H}{\partial R^*}\frac{R^*}{H}\frac{dR^*}{dE}\frac{1}{R^*} + \frac{\partial H}{\partial Q^*}\frac{Q^*}{H}\frac{dQ^*}{dE}\frac{1}{Q^*}$$

$$\hat{H} = \eta_H\frac{d\ln R^*}{dE} - e_H\frac{d\ln Q^*}{dE}.$$

Since $\ln R^* = \ln R - \ln Q$ and since R is fixed,

$$\frac{d\ln R^*}{dE} = -\frac{d\ln Q}{dE} = r_E$$

$$\frac{d\ln Q^*}{dE} = \frac{d\ln \pi}{dE} - \frac{d\ln Q}{dE} = -r_H + r_E.$$

Hence,

$$\hat{H} = r_E\eta_H + e_H(r_H - r_E).$$ (C-10)

Since $\hat{M} = \hat{H} - r_H$, the human capital parameter in the demand curve for medical care would be

$$\hat{M} = r_E(\eta_H - 1) + (r_H - r_E)(e_H - 1).$$ (C-11)

Appendix D

STATISTICAL PROPERTIES
OF THE MODEL

1. STRUCTURE AND REDUCED FORM

Let the demand curve for the stock of health be given by

$$\ln H_i = \varepsilon \ln W_i - \varepsilon \ln \pi_i - \varepsilon \ln (r - \tilde{\pi}_i + \delta_i), \qquad \text{(D-1)}$$

the depreciation rate function by

$$\ln \delta_i = \ln \delta_0 + \tilde{\delta} i, \qquad \text{(D-2)}$$

and the gross investment production function by

$$\ln I_i = r_H E + \alpha_1 \ln M_i + (1 - \alpha_1) \ln TH_i, \qquad \text{(D-3)}$$

where all variables are expressed as deviations from their respective means. Substituting (D-2) into (D-1) and assuming that $r - \tilde{\pi}_i = 0$, one gets

$$\ln H_i = \varepsilon \ln W_i - \varepsilon \ln \pi_i - \tilde{\delta} \varepsilon i - \varepsilon \ln \delta_0. \qquad \text{(D-4)}$$

The total cost of gross investment can be written

$$C_i = \pi_i I_i = PM_i + W_i TH_i, \qquad \text{(D-5)}$$

and in least-cost equilibrium

$$\frac{g - tg'}{g'} = \frac{P}{W_i} = \frac{\alpha_1}{1 - \alpha_1} \frac{TH_i}{M_i}. \qquad \text{(D-6)}$$

Utilization of (D-3), (D-5), and (D-6) gives the marginal cost function

$$\ln \pi_i = K \ln W_i + (1 - K) \ln P - r_H E, \qquad \text{(D-7)}$$

where $K = 1 - \alpha_1$ and $1 - K = \alpha_1$. Substitution of equation (D-7) into equation (D-4) generates the reduced form demand curve for the stock of health.

$$\ln H_i = (1 - K)\varepsilon \ln W_i - (1 - K)\varepsilon \ln P + r_H \varepsilon E - \tilde{\delta} \varepsilon i - \varepsilon \ln \delta_0. \quad \text{(D-8)}$$

Having obtained a stock demand curve, one can proceed to calculate a derived demand curve for medical care. If the production function equation is solved for $\ln M_i$, then

$$\ln M_i = \alpha_1^{-1} \ln I_i - (1 - \alpha_1)\alpha_1^{-1} \ln TH_i - \alpha_1^{-1} r_H E.$$

But $\ln I_i = \ln H_i + \ln(\tilde{H}_i + \delta_i)$. Hence,

$$\ln M_i = \alpha_1^{-1} \ln H_i + \alpha_1^{-1} \ln(\tilde{H}_i + \delta_i) - (1 - \alpha_1)\alpha_1^{-1} \ln TH_i - \alpha_1^{-1} r_H E.$$

Equations (D-6) and (D-8) can be employed to show that an alternative form of the last equation is

$$\ln M_i = [(1 - K)\varepsilon + K] \ln W_i - [(1 - K)\varepsilon + K] \ln P + r_E(\varepsilon - 1)E$$
$$- \tilde{\delta}\varepsilon i - \varepsilon \ln \delta_0 + \ln(\tilde{H} + \delta_i).$$

The last term on the right-hand side of this equation can be rewritten as $\ln \delta_i + \ln(1 + \tilde{H}_i/\delta_i)$. From (D-2),

$$\ln \delta_i + \ln(1 + \tilde{H}/\delta_i) = \ln \delta_0 + \tilde{\delta}i + \ln(1 + \tilde{H}_i/\delta_i).$$

Therefore, the reduced form demand curve for medical care is

$$\ln M_i = [(1 - K)\varepsilon + K] \ln W_i - [(1 - K)\varepsilon + K] \ln P + r_E(\varepsilon - 1)E$$
$$+ \tilde{\delta}(1 - \varepsilon)i + (1 - \varepsilon) \ln \delta_0 + \ln(1 + \tilde{H}/\delta_i). \tag{D-9}$$

2. THE EFFECTS OF ERRORS OF MEASUREMENT

Suppose P does not vary across the relevant units of observation, $\tilde{H}_i/\delta_i$ is small, and wealth is excluded from the set of exogenous variables.[1] Then the reduced form would be

$$\ln H_i = B_1 + B_W \ln \overline{W} + B_E E' + B_i i + u_1 \tag{D-10}$$

$$\ln M_i = B_2 + B_{WM} \ln \overline{W} + B_{EM} E' + B_i i + u_2, \tag{D-11}$$

where $\overline{W}$ is the true wage at age i and E' is a measure of efficiency in non-market production. The investment model predicts $B_W > 0$, $B_{E'} > 0$, $B_i < 0$, and $B_{WM} > 0$. In addition, if $\varepsilon < 1$, $B_{E'M} < 0$ and $B_{iM} > 0$. The problem of errors of measurement arises in estimating these equations for two reasons. First, at any given age, a person's observed wage may contain a transitory component due to factors such as unexpected unemployment

[1] The analysis of errors of measurement would be considerably more complicated if wealth or family income were one of the independent variables. None of the basic conclusions reached in this section, however, would be substantially altered.

and response errors. Second, the variable E' in (D-10) and (D-11) is not education per se. Instead, it is a more general index of efficiency in non-market production. This index depends on education, E, but also depends on a vector of other variables, u_3, that reflects variations in nonmarket ability across individuals with the same amount of formal schooling.

Let the relation between the true wage and the observed (measured) wage be

$$\ln \overline{W} = \ln W - \ln W^*, \tag{D-12}$$

where $\ln W^*$ is the transitory component. In addition, let the equation for nonmarket efficiency be

$$E' = a_1 + a_2 E + a_3 u_3, \tag{D-13}$$

where $a_2 > 0$ and $a_3 > 0$. Substitution of (D-12) and (D-13) into (D-10), yields

$$H = B_1 + B_E a_1 + B_W W + B_E a_2 E + B_i i + u_1 - B_W W^* + B_E a_3 u_3$$

or

$$H = B_1^* + B_W W + B_E E + B_i i + u_4, \tag{D-14}$$

where $u_4 = u_1 - B_W W^* + B_E a_3 u_3$.[2] If (D-14) is fitted by ordinary least squares, the estimated equation would be

$$H = b_1 + b_W W + b_E E + b_i i + e,$$

or in matrix notation

$$H = Xb + e.$$

To determine whether the regression coefficients in the vector b are unbiased estimates of the true population parameters, write

$$b = (X'X)^{-1} X'H.$$

The expected value of this vector is

$$E(b) = E[(X'X)^{-1} X'(XB + u_4)]$$
$$E(b) = B + (X'X)^{-1} E(X'u_4).$$

---

[2] The abbreviation for natural logarithm, ln, is omitted before H, W, $\overline{W}$, and W^* from now on.

Note that $(X'X)^{-1} = \sigma^2 b/\sigma^2 u_4$. Note also that

$$(X'X)^{-1} = \begin{bmatrix} K_W & -r_{WE}K_{WE} & -r_{Wi}K_{Wi} \\ -r_{EW}K_{EW} & +K_E & -r_{Ei}K_{Ei} \\ -r_{iW}K_{iW} & -r_{iE}K_{iE} & +K_i \end{bmatrix} \qquad \text{(D-16)}$$

where, for example, $K_W = \sigma^2 b_W/\sigma^2 u_4 > 0$, $K_{WE} = (\sigma b_W \sigma b_E/\sigma^2 u_4) > 0$, and r_{WE} is the partial correlation coefficient between W and E, with i held constant.[3] Thus, the sign of a typical off-diagonal element in $(X'X)^{-1}$ depends solely on the partial correlation between the two relevant independent variables.

Equation (D-16) allows one to compare the expected value of any regression coefficient with its true value. For instance, the term in the matrix $E(b)$ that corresponds to the regression coefficient of the wage rate is

$$E(b_W) = B_W + K_W E[\text{Cov}(Wu_4)] - r_{WE}K_{WE}E[\text{Cov}(Eu_4)]$$
$$- r_{Wi}K_{Wi}E[\text{Cov}(iu_4)].$$

To determine the biases introduced by errors of measurement, the correlation between u_4 and each of the independent variables must be evaluated. It is reasonable to suppose that age and education are independent of u_4. It is also reasonable to assume that the wage rate is positively correlated with u_3 because *market* and *nonmarket* ability are positively correlated. In other words, an increase in u_3, with education held constant, reflects an increase in nonmarket efficiency. On the other hand, an increase in the wage, with age and education fixed, may be viewed as an increase in market efficiency. Then if W^* were independent of $\overline{W}$,

$$E[\text{Cov}(Eu_4)] = E[\text{Cov}(iu_4)] = 0$$
$$E[\text{Cov}(Wu_4)] = -B_W\sigma^2 W^* + B_E a_3 \text{Cov}(Wu_3),$$

and

$$E(b_W) = B_W - K_E B_W\sigma^2 W^* + K_W B_E a_3 \text{Cov}(Wu_3)$$
$$E(b_E) = B_E + r_{EW}K_{EW}B_W\sigma^2 W^* - r_{EW}K_{EW}B_E a_3 \text{Cov}(Wu_3) \qquad \text{(D-17)}$$
$$E(b_i) = B_i + r_{iW}K_{iW}B_W\sigma^2 W^* - r_{iW}K_{iW}B_E a_3 \text{Cov}(Wu_3).$$

[3] For a derivation of equation (D-16), see Yoel Haitovsky, "Simplified Formulae for Covariance B," New York, NBER, mimeographed, 1968. See also Robert T. Michael, *The Effect of Education on Efficiency in Consumption*, New York, NBER, Occasional Paper 116, 1972, Appendix B. Much of my discussion of the effects of errors of measurement is based on Michael's formulation of the problem.

Equation (D-17) suggests that two types of biases operate on the estimated coefficients. The first is due to measurement error in the wage variable and is represented by the variance of the transitory wage, $\sigma^2 W^*$. The second is due to the positive correlation between market and non-market ability and is represented by the term $\text{Cov}(Wu_3)$. Since $B_W > 0$, the presence of random errors of observation biases the wage coefficient downward. Since $B_E a_3 > 0$ and $\text{Cov}(Wu_3) > 0$, the ability effect biases this coefficient upward. So the net impact of these two biases on the wage coefficient is not certain.

In the NORC sample, $r_{EW} = .418$ and $r_{iW} = .135$.[4] Since both these partial correlation coefficients are positive, measurement error biases the age and education coefficients upward, while ability biases them downward. Consequently, the important conclusion is reached that none of the coefficients in the demand curve for health is biased in an *obvious* direction.

The situation is very different in the demand curve for medical care. In that demand curve, the expected value of the regression coefficient of education—or of nonmarket ability in general—would be negative if the elasticity of the MEC schedule were less than unity. Given this condition, both the measurement error and the ability effects would bias the wage coefficient *downward*. Moreover, both these effects would bias the education and age coefficients *upward*. The important point to stress is that the two sources of bias operate in *opposite* directions on any given coefficient in the demand curve for health but operate in the *same* direction on the corresponding coefficient in the demand curve for medical care.

---

[4] These partial correlations pertain to whites with positive sick time. They hold constant sex and family size as well as age or education.

Appendix E

ADDITIONAL EMPIRICAL RESULTS

1. A PRIORI ESTIMATES

The observed effects of education and the wage rate on the demand for health reported in Chapter V are precisely the ones predicted by the investment model. The coefficients of these two variables have the "wrong signs," however, in the demand curve for medical care. Appendix D showed that biases introduced by (1) measurement error in the wage rate and (2) a positive association between the wage and innate ability operate in opposite directions on a given health regression coefficient but in the same direction on the corresponding medical care coefficient. Since the two sources of bias tend to offset each other in the health demand curve, it is not surprising that the estimates of its parameters are more consistent with a priori notions. Moreover, the correlation between the wage rate and education exceeds the correlation between the former and any of the other independent variables except income. So the negative relation between the wage rate and the medical care function's error term seriously affects not only the estimate of the wage elasticity but also the estimate of the education parameter.[1]

Assuming that the biases exactly offset each other in the health demand function, one can use its education or wage coefficient to solve for the corresponding medical care coefficient. He can then force the education coefficient, for example, to assume its proper value and examine the effect of this procedure on the estimates of the other coefficients of the medical care demand curve. In the stock of health demand curve in Table 1, the education coefficient is $r_H\varepsilon = .025$. Since $\varepsilon = .5$, $r_H = .05$. Therefore, education's medical care parameter should be $r_H(\varepsilon - 1) = -.025$. Consequently, if $\ln M + .025E$ were the dependent variable in the medical care demand function and if E were excluded from the regression, its coefficient would be forced to equal the appropriate value.

---

[1] The difficult question of the effect of the biases on the income elasticity of medical care was not treated in Appendix D. This appendix comments on the change in the income elasticity induced by improved estimates of the wage and education parameters.

Along similar lines, the stock elasticity of the wage rate is $(1 - K)\varepsilon = .090$, which suggests $K = .82$.[2] The wage elasticity of medical care is given by $(1 - K)\varepsilon + K\sigma_p$, where σ_p is the elasticity of substitution between medical care and own time in the production of gross investment. The Cobb-Douglas specification implies $\sigma_p = 1$, so the wage elasticity of medical care should equal .910. By defining the dependent variable as $\ln M - .910 \ln W$ and excluding $\ln W$ from the regression, such a value would actually be obtained. The structure and reduced form of the model would be practically unaffected if medical care and own time were employed in fixed proportions. Therefore, σ_p might also be set equal to zero to get a lower bound on the wage elasticity. In this case, the elasticity would be .090, and the dependent variable in the medical care demand curve would be $\ln M - .090 \ln W$.

Table E-1 gives demand curves for medical care that take account of the a priori restrictions on the coefficients of E and $\ln W$. In the first regression in Part A of the table, the coefficient of E is set equal to $-.025$. In the second, the wage elasticity equals .910, while in the third, it equals .090. The fourth regression defines the dependent variable as $\ln M + .025E - .910 \ln W$ so that both restrictions are imposed simultaneously. Finally, the fifth regression uses $\ln M + .025E - .090 \ln W$ as the dependent variable.

The regressions in Part B of the table are based on the coefficients of E and $\ln W$ in the health flow demand curve.[3] This function suggests that education's medical care parameter should be $-.046$. It also suggests a wage elasticity of .676 if $\sigma_p = 1$ and an elasticity of .324 if $\sigma_p = 0$.

The table shows that when the education coefficient alone is restricted, the wage elasticity increases in absolute value. In Table 3, this elasticity equals $-.105$, in Part A of Table E-1 it equals $-.009$, and in Part B, it equals .046. Although the wage elasticity is still negative in Part A and is never statistically significant, the magnitude of its increase is substantial.

Restricted wage elasticities that are based on an elasticity of substitution equal to unity make the education coefficient negative but not statistically significant. These wage elasticities generate income elasticities equal to .080 (Part A) and .221 (Part B). Such elasticities are smaller than

---

[2] In this section, all wage elasticities of health are taken from regressions that use $Y4$ as the income variable. These elasticities give conservative lower estimates of the true parameters.

[3] In particular, averages of the wage and education coefficients in the work-loss days and restricted-activity days regressions are used.

TABLE E-1

A Priori Estimates of Demand for Medical Care by Whites with Positive Sick Time

Assumed σ_p	ln $Y4$	ln W	E	i	Sex	ln FS	$\bar{R}^2$
A. Based on Stock Coefficients							
Not restricted	.685	−.009	−.025[a]	.013	.548	−.222	.073
	(3.86)	(−.05)		(2.41)	(2.82)	(−1.41)	
1	.080	.910[a]	−.035	.014	1.024	−.020	.072
	(.56)		(−1.51)	(2.35)	(5.78)	(−.13)	
0	.576	.090[a]	.002	.016	.600	−.168	·067
	(4.17)		(.11)	(2.67)	(3.47)	(−1.09)	
1	.064	.910[a]	−.025[a]	.015	1.025	−.009	.069
	(.46)			(2.56)	(5.79)	(−.06)	
0	.618	.090[a]	−.025[a]	.014	.599	−.199	.070
	(4.61)			(2.43)	(3.49)	(−1.31)	
B. Based on Flow Coefficients							
Not restricted´	.680	.046	−.046[a]	.012	.576	−.232	.075
	(3.82)	(.27)		(2.16)	(2.95)	(−1.47)	
1	.221	.676[a]	−.024	.014	.903	−.062	.063
	(1.58)		(−1.06)	(2.45)	(5.15)	(−.50)	
0	.435	.324[a]	−.008	.015	.721	−.126	.061
	(3.13)		(−.36)	(2.58)	(4.16)	(−.82)	
1	.254	.676[a]	−.046[a]	.013	.902	−.086	.063
	(1.87)			(2.28)	(5.15)	(−.56)	
0	.492	.324[a]	−.046[a]	.012	.720	−.168	.064
	(3.65)			(2.22)	(4.15)	(−1.10)	

[a] Coefficient *forced* to assume the value shown.

all existing estimates, and few students of the demand for medical care would accept their validity.[4] More reasonable income elasticities result when σ_p is set equal to zero, particularly when the education coefficient is

[4] Previous studies indicate that the income elasticity of medical care is slightly less than unity. If the wage elasticity is positive, then these estimates are biased upward. In a recent study, Morris Silver computed an income elasticity that did hold the wage rate constant. He obtained an income elasticity of 1.20 and a wage elasticity of 2.07. (See "An Economic Analysis of Variations in Medical Expenses and Work-Loss Rates," in Herbert E. Klarman (ed.), *Empirical Studies in Health Economics*, Baltimore, 1970, and reprinted as Chapter 6 in Victor R. Fuchs (ed.), *Essays in the Economics of Health and Medical Care*, New York, NBER, 1972. In my judgment, Silver's elasticities are unreasonably high.

also constrained to be negative. If the wage coefficient alone is restricted and is assumed to equal .090, the education coefficient falls from .012 (Table 3) to .002 (Table E-1, Part A). While education still has a positive effect on medical care in the a priori demand curve, the size of this effect is much smaller.

The conclusions to be drawn from a priori estimation are, at best, tentative because the technique assumes that the health coefficients are unbiased. But the results do indicate that an a priori computation of the education parameter improves the actual estimate of the wage elasticity. Conversely, an a priori computation of the wage elasticity improves the actual estimate of the education parameter. The reduction in the calculated education effect and the increase in the wage effect suggest that biases introduced by errors of measurement may play an important role in the demand curve for medical care. The results also indicate that the elasticity of substitution between medical care and own time is small. This means that even if the wage elasticity is positive, it cannot be very large.

2. DEMAND CURVES: ALL WHITES IN THE LABOR FORCE, MALES, AND FEMALES

Tables E-2, E-3, and E-4 present a complete set of demand curves for all whites in the labor force. Tables E-5, E-6, and E-7 present a complete set of these functions for males with positive sick time; and Tables E-8, E-9, and E-10 give demand curves for females with positive sick time. The reader is left to inspect these tables for himself.

TABLE E-2

Stock Demand for Health by All Whites in the Labor Force

Income Measure	ln Y	ln W	E	i	Sex	ln FS	$\bar{R}^2$
Y1	.006	.067	.022	−.007	−.036	−.027	.106
	(.26)	(3.15)	(6.83)	(−8.54)	(−1.43)	(−1.20)	
Y2	.015	.062	.022	−.007	−.034	−.030	.106
	(.61)	(2.92)	(6.85)	(−8.56)	(−1.52)	(−1.30)	
Y4	.019	.060	.022	−.007	−.041	−.032	.106
	(.84)	(2.96)	(6.76)	(−8.56)	(−1.58)	(−1.37)	
Y4	.057		.025	−.007	−.080	−.043	.102
	(3.00)		(7.58)	(−8.39)	(−3.60)	(−1.87)	
Y omitted		.070	.022	−.007	−.035	−.026	.106
		(1.11)	(6.96)	(8.55)	(1.10)	(1.17)	

NOTE: The health stock series is 1 = poor, 2 = fair, 3 = good, 6 = excellent.

TABLE E-3
Flow Demand for Health by All Whites in the Labor Force

Income Measure	ln $Y4$	ln W	E	i	Sex	ln FS	$\bar{R}^2$
			$TL = WLD1$				
$Y1$	.048	.207	.066	−.009	.114	.180	.008
	(.26)	(1.25)	(2.52)	(−1.23)	(.57)	(1.02)	
$Y2$	−.128	.295	.066	−.009	.163	.220	.008
	(−.66)	(1.80)	(2.66)	(−1.17)	(.80)	(1.23)	
$Y4$	−.092	.277	.066	−.009	.150	.216	.008
	(−.52)	(1.75)	(2.65)	(−1.18)	(.75)	(1.20)	
$Y4$	.079		.079	−.009	−.031	.163	.007
	(.55)		(3.11)	(−1.07)	(−.17)	(.92)	
Y omitted		.229	.066	−.009	.123	.185	.009
		(1.76)	(2.60)	(−1.22)	(.63)	(1.09)	
			$TL = RAD$				
$Y1$	−.132	.066	.054	−.006	−.222	.282	.004
	(−.67)	(.38)	(2.02)	(−.92)	(−1.09)	(1.56)	
$Y2$	−.300	.150	.054	−.006	−.156	.336	.005
	(−1.45)	(.86)	(2.09)	(−.88)	(−.72)	(1.80)	
$Y4$	−.294	.144	.060	−.006	−.156	.348	.005
	(−1.56)	(.85)	(2.15)	(−.87)	(−.75)	(1.87)	
$Y4$	−.204		.060	−.006	−.252	.324	.005
	(−1.31)		(2.40)	(−.82)	(−1.38)	(1.75)	
Y omitted		−.006	.048	−.006	−.252	.264	.004
		(−.02)	(1.93)	(−.97)	(−1.23)	(1.46)	

TABLE E-4
Demand for Medical Care by All Whites in the Labor Force

Income Measure	ln Y	ln W	E	i	Sex	ln FS	$\bar{R}^2$
$Y1$	.450	.036	.026	.012	.585	−.197	.039
	(3.79)	(.35)	(1.60)	(3.04)	(4.72)	(−1.80)	
$Y2$	.548	−.008	.027	.012	.495	−.257	.042
	(4.44)	(−.07)	(1.74)	(3.04)	(3.86)	(−2.30)	
$Y4$	.521	.014	.025	.012	.507	−.280	.043
	(4.66)	(.14)	(1.53)	(3.03)	(4.01)	(−2.48)	
$Y4$	.530		.025	.012	.499	−.282	.043
	(5.71)		(1.60)	(3.04)	(4.59)	(−2.54)	
Y omitted		.272	.036	.013	.670	−.122	.032
		(3.28)	(2.25)	(3.30)	(5.47)	(−1.13)	

TABLE E-5
Stock Demand for Health by Males with Positive Sick Time

Income Measure	ln Y	ln W	E	i	ln FS	$\bar{R}^2$
Y1	.040	.106	.028	−.010	.018	.193
	(.63)	(1.69)	(4.01)	(−5.89)	(.41)	
Y2	.041	.109	.028	−.010	.018	.193
	(.70)	(1.95)	(4.03)	(−5.90)	(.40)	
Y4	.041	.111	.028	−.010	.017	.193
	(.76)	(2.13)	(4.01)	(−5.89)	(.38)	
Y4	.118		.033	−.009	.010	.186
	(2.90)		(5.13)	(−5.73)	(.22)	
Y omitted		.138	.028	−.010	.019	.194
		(3.53)	(3.98)	(−5.87)	(.43)	

NOTE: The health stock series is 1 = poor, 1.6 = fair, 2.9 = good, 4.9 = excellent.

TABLE E-6
Flow Demand for Health by Males with Positive Sick Time

Income Measure	ln Y	ln W	E	i	ln FS	$\bar{R}^2$
			$TL = WLD1$			
Y1	−.324	.660	.050	−.012	.318	.125
	(−1.88)	(3.87)	(2.65)	(−2.62)	(2.68)	
Y2	−.289	.606	.048	−.012	.319	.125
	(−1.80)	(3.99)	(2.57)	(−2.61)	(2.69)	
Y4	−.040	.434	.052	−.012	.314	.118
	(−.27)	(3.06)	(2.77)	(−2.69)	(2.63)	
Y4	.260		.073	−.011	.287	.099
	(2.34)		(4.14)	(−2.45)	(2.39)	
Y omitted		.409	.052	−.012	.312	.120
		(3.87)	(2.79)	(−2.71)	(2.62)	
			$TL = RAD$			
Y1	−.340	.515	.045	−.014	.257	.088
	(−1.91)	(2.92)	(2.31)	(−3.01)	(2.10)	
Y2	−.292	.450	.044	−.014	.258	.087
	(−1.76)	(2.87)	(2.24)	(−3.01)	(2.10)	
Y4	−.138	.339	.047	−.014	.257	.082
	(−.91)	(2.32)	(2.40)	(−3.06)	(2.09)	
Y4	.096		.063	−.013	.236	.072
	(.84)		(3.48)	(−2.89)	(1.91)	
Y omitted		.251	.048	−.014	.251	.082
		(2.30)	(2.46)	(−3.19)	(2.04)	

TABLE E-7

Demand for Medical Care by Males with Positive Sick Time

Income Measure	ln Y	ln W	E	i	ln FS	$\bar{R}^2$
Y1	.857	−.477	.028	.025	−.294	.071
	(3.24)	(−1.83)	(.97)	(3.74)	(−1.62)	
Y2	.934	−.449	.034	.025	−.301	.080
	(3.83)	(−1.94)	(1.18)	(3.70)	(−1.67)	
Y4	.869	−.369	.027	.025	−.314	.082
	(3.92)	(−1.73)	(.94)	(3.76)	(−1.75)	
Y4	.618		.009	.025	−.293	.077
	(3.70)		(.32)	(3.63)	(−1.62)	
Y omitted		.188	.021	.026	−.278	.049
		(1.15)	(.71)	(3.86)	(−1.51)	

TABLE E-8

Stock Demand for Health by Females with Positive Sick Time

($N = 152$)

Income Measure	ln Y	ln W	E	i	ln FS	$\bar{R}^2$
Y1	−.086	.130	.013	−.004	.035	.006
	(−.80)	(1.21)	(.98)	(−1.14)	(.40)	
Y2	.046	.051	.011	−.005	−.024	.003
	(.40)	(.46)	(.85)	(−1.38)	(−.23)	
Y4	.110	.009	.011	−.005	−.071	.010
	(1.10)	(.08)	(.84)	(−1.52)	(−.68)	
Y4	.116		.011	−.005	−.075	.016
	(1.44)		(.89)	(−1.53)	(−.79)	
Y omitted		.080	.011	−.004	[a]	.015
		(.92)	(.88)	(−1.38)		

NOTE: The health stock series is 1 = poor, 1.8 = fair, 1.6 = good, 5.1 = excellent.

[a] The variable was deleted by the regression program since its F ratio was less than .005.

TABLE E-9
Flow Demand for Health by Females with Positive Sick Time

Income Measure	ln Y	ln W	E	i	ln FS	$\bar{R}^2$
			$TL = WLD1$			
Y1	−.193	.228	.039	.008	.080	−.011
	(−.77)	(.90)	(1.24)	(1.04)	(.38)	
Y2	.097	.053	.035	.007	−.049	−.014
	(.36)	(.20)	(1.12)	(.82)	(−.20)	
Y4	.184	−.004	.034	.006	−.115	−.010
	(.78)	(−.02)	(1.11)	(.74)	(−.47)	
Y4	.182		.034	.006	−.114	−.004
	(.96)		(1.15)	(.74)	(−.51)	
Y omitted		.113	.035	.007	a	−.001
		(.56)	(1.15)	(.91)		
			$TL = RAD$			
Y1	−.223	.082	.050	.006	.144	−.015
	(−.85)	(.30)	(1.52)	(.70)	(.66)	
Y2	−.091	.005	.046	.005	.117	−.019
	(−.32)	(.02)	(1.42)	(.58)	(.45)	
Y4	−.099	.011	.046	.005	.129	−.019
	(−.40)	(.04)	(1.42)	(.60)	(.50)	
Y4	−.093		.047	.005	.124	−.012
	(−.46)		(1.48)	(.60)	(.53)	
Y omitted		−.052	.046	.004	.062	−.013
		(−.24)	(1.41)	(.54)	(.32)	

a The variable was deleted by the regression program since its F ratio was less than .005.

TABLE E-10
Demand for Medical Care by Females with Positive Sick Time

Income Measure	ln Y	ln W	E	i	ln FS	$\bar{R}^2$
Y1	.518	.354	−.019	−.002	.077	.027
	(1.51)	(1.03)	(−.45)	(−.18)	(.27)	
Y2	.409	.405	−.012	−.001	.019	.020
	(1.13)	(1.12)	(−.27)	(−.06)	(.06)	
Y4	.349	.437	−.011	−.001	.028	.019
	(1.08)	(1.26)	(−.26)	(−.07)	(.08)	
Y4	.590		.003	−.001	−.144	.015
	(2.27)		(.08)	(−.06)	(−.47)	
Y omitted		.661	−.009	.001	.265	.018
		(2.36)	(−.22)	(.13)	(1.04)	

Appendix F

SOURCES AND METHODS: MORTALITY ANALYSIS

The purpose of this appendix is to discuss the sources and definitions of the variables used in the regression analysis for states of the United States. All variables except average hourly earnings of paramedical personnel and the price of cigarettes pertain to whites only.

(1) *State population distributions by age and sex*, 1960: U.S. Department of Commerce, Bureau of the Census, *1960 Census of Population*, Volume I: *Characteristics of the Population*, Summary Volume, Table 59 and State Volumes, Table 94. Hereafter cited as COP.

(2) *Expected death rate*: Let $\bar{d}_j$ be the expected death rate in the jth state, F_j be the population of that state, and F_{isj} be the number of people in an age-sex cell in that state. Also let d_{isUS} be a U.S. age-sex specific death rate. Then

$$\bar{d}_j = \sum_{i=1}^{11} \sum_{s=1}^{2} d_{isUS} F_{isj} / F_j.$$

The eleven age cells used in this computation are : <1, 1–4, 5–14, 15–24, 25–34, 35–44, 45–54, 55–64, 65–74, 75–84, and 85+.

(3) *Crude death rate*: U.S. Department of Health, Education and Welfare, Public Health Service, National Vital Statistics Division, *Vital Statistics of the United States*, Volume II: *Mortality, 1959–61*, selected tables. The crude death rate is defined as a three-year average of death rates for the years 1959, 1960, and 1961.

(4) *Median income of families and unrelated individuals*, 1959: COP, State Volumes, Table 65.

(5) *Earnings*, 1959: COP, State Volumes, Table 130. Median earnings are available separately for males and females, but data without a sex break are not available. Instead of combining the two distributions of earnings and calculating a median for the entire labor force, I weighted median earnings of males and females by the proportion of each group in the experienced civilian labor force. Sample calculations indicate that this method yields almost the same results as the first. Observe that earnings and income were not adjusted for variations in weeks worked because the number of weeks worked is practically constant across states. Observe

also that these two variables were not adjusted for net earnings lost due to work-loss because there are no data that measure this variable for states.

(6) *Education*, 1960: COP, State Volumes, Table 47. Education is defined as the median number of years of formal schooling completed by the population 25 years of age and above.

(7) *Price of paramedical personnel*, 1959: Richard D. Auster, Irving Leveson, and Deborah Sarachek, "The Production of Health, an Exploratory Study," *Journal of Human Resources*, 4, No. 4 (Fall 1969), and reprinted as Chapter 8 in Victor R. Fuchs (ed.), *Essays in the Economics of Health and Medical Care*, New York, NBER, 1972, Table G-1. This variable is defined as the ratio of actual to expected hourly earnings as shown in the 1/1,000 sample.[1] Since persons in the sample were not classified by state, Auster, Leveson, and Sarachek computed this variable for two occupations (professional nurses and all other paramedical personnel) by region (Northeast, North Central, South, and West) and by residence (inside SMSA and outside SMSA). State estimates by occupation were obtained by classifying the states according to region and then averaging the region's ratio of actual to expected earnings using as weights the proportion of paramedical employment in each occupation.

(8) *Price of cigarettes*: Tobacco Tax Council, *The Tax Burden on Tobacco: Historical Compilation* (1966), Table 13. The price used is an average for the years 1959–61. Federal and state cigarette taxes are included in this price, but municipal taxes are excluded.

---

[1] The expected hourly earnings of a given person is that earnings figure that would be predicted if the person had the same earnings as all U.S. nonagricultural employed individuals with the same age, sex, color, and education characteristics. For a complete description, see Victor R. Fuchs, *Differentials in Hourly Earnings by Region and City Size, 1959*, New York, NBER, Occasional Paper 101, 1967.

INDEX